T0249673

Nanoparticles and the Immune System

Nanoparticles and the Immune System
Safety and Effects

Diana Boraschi and Albert Duschl

AMSTERDAM • BOSTON • HEIDELBERG • LONDON
NEW YORK • OXFORD • PARIS • SAN DIEGO
SAN FRANCISCO • SINGAPORE • SYDNEY • TOKYO
Academic Press is an imprint of Elsevier

Academic Press is an imprint of Elsevier
The Boulevard, Langford Lane, Kidlington, Oxford, OX5 1GB, UK
225 Wyman Street, Waltham, MA 02451, USA

First published 2014

Copyright © 2014 Elsevier Inc. All rights reserved

No part of this publication may be reproduced or transmitted in any form or by any
means, electronic or mechanical, including photocopying, recording, or any information
storage and retrieval system, without permission in writing from the publisher. Details on
how to seek permission, further information about the Publisher's permissions policies
and our arrangement with organizations such as the Copyright Clearance Center and the
Copyright Licensing Agency, can be found at our website: www.elsevier.com/permissions.

This book and the individual contributions contained in it are protected under
copyright by the Publisher (other than as may be noted herein).

Notices
Knowledge and best practice in this field are constantly changing. As new research
and experience broaden our understanding, changes in research methods, professional
practices, or medical treatment may become necessary.

Practitioners and researchers must always rely on their own experience and knowledge
in evaluating and using any information, methods, compounds, or experiments described
herein. In using such information or methods they should be mindful of their own safety
and the safety of others, including parties for whom they have a professional
responsibility.

To the fullest extent of the law, neither the Publisher nor the authors, contributors,
or editors, assume any liability for any injury and/or damage to persons or property
as a matter of products liability, negligence or otherwise, or from any use or operation
of any methods, products, instructions, or ideas contained in the material herein.

British Library Cataloguing-in-Publication Data
A catalogue record for this book is available from the British Library

Library of Congress Cataloging-in-Publication Data
A catalog record for this book is available from the Library of Congress

ISBN: 978-0-12-408085-0

For information on all Academic Press publications
visit our website at **store.elsevier.com**

This book has been manufactured using Print On Demand technology. Each copy
is produced to order and is limited to black ink. The online version of this book
will show color figures where appropriate.

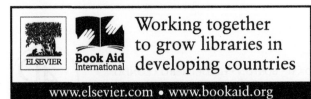

Working together
to grow libraries in
developing countries

www.elsevier.com • www.bookaid.org

CONTENTS

PREFACE

This book has the objective to provide a reference text for toxicologists, materials scientists, and regulators by covering the key issues that define interaction of nanomaterials with the immune system. Altering immune responses can lead to many kinds of pathologies; therefore, it is important to make adequate assessments before new nanomaterials are introduced in the market. On the other hand, negative perception and excessive concerns, based on incomplete or misleading results, need to be avoided by communicating existing knowledge and by defining in the future clear endpoints and thresholds for immunosafety regulations.

Nanotoxicology investigations often focus on toxicity leading to death of cells or organisms, while important immune parameters can be affected much earlier and at much lower doses. Some aspects of immunity, for example allergic sensitivity and heightened danger for risk persons with a frail immune system, are usually not covered at all. This gap in nanosafety assessment needs to be filled, not only from a scientific point of view but also for a better implementation of relevant safety regulations. A friend and nanotoxicologist, Jan Mats, told us once: "if we do not consider immunity, we keep studying the mouse without seeing the elephant in the room." To increase the awareness of the importance of immunity in nanotoxicology, several years ago we started the Immunosafety Focus Group within the Working Group "Hazard" of the EU-supported NanoSafety Cluster, and this book intends to disseminate knowledge gained by the research community in this field.

The book covers several issues that all stakeholders in nanotechnology should be aware of: identification of endpoints that are relevant for assessing hazard, evaluating impact on immunologically frail populations, considering allergic responses, and how to evaluate chronic/cumulative effects. In addition, the book addresses a very important issue, that is, how to shape and turn the immunomodulating properties of nanomaterials to our advantage for preventive strategies (such as vaccination) or for therapeutic approaches in diseases where immunostimulation is desired (infections, tumors) or where immunosuppression in needed (inflammatory diseases, allergies, autoimmunity).

Our goal is to raise awareness about the effects of nanomaterials on our immune system, in order to ensure a safe design or safe use of such materials. We also want to emphasize an especially useful role of the immune system: it has been optimized by evolution to identify whether or not specific foreign materials are dangerous to the body. Finding that out is also the key question in nanosafety, so knowing the opinion of the professional immune cells should be of particular interest to us.

Diana Boraschi and Albert Duschl

ACKNOWLEDGMENTS

The editors Diana Boraschi and Albert Duschl wish to thank the many individuals who have stimulated them in various occasions (publications, presentations at congresses, personal discussions) to put the immune response toward nanomaterials into the general context of immunity. We thank our working groups for giving us input on many questions and for being patient when we were unavailable due to intense work on the book. Most of all, we thank our partners, Aldo and Jutta, who have supported us with their patience and attention, and who granted us the time to work on this book.

The research leading to this book has received support from the European Union Seventh Framework Programme (FP7/2007–2013) projects NanoEIS (NMP-2012-CSA-6-GA 319054; AD), NanoValid (NMP-2010-1.3-1-GA 263147; AD), NanoTOES (PITN-GA-2010-2645506; AD and DB), NANoREG (NMP-LA-2013-310584; DB), HUMUNITY (PITN-GA-2012-316383; DB), and QualityNano (INFRA-2010-262163; DB).

Albert Duschl gratefully acknowledges support from the research cluster "Biosciences and Health" of the University of Salzburg.

Diana Boraschi gratefully acknowledges the support from the Fondazione Cariplo within the project "Inter-cellular delivery, trafficking and toxicity of engineered magnetic nanoparticles in macrophages and CNS cells."

S. Moein Moghimi gratefully acknowledges the support by the Danish Agency for Science, Technology and Innovation (Det Strategiske Forskningsråd), reference 09-065746.

Laura Canesi wishes to thank Caterina Ciacci (University of Urbino, Italy) and Rita Fabbri (University of Genoa, Italy) for their invaluable technical assistance in the experimental work on nanoparticles and mussel immunocytes, and Gabriella Gallo for her foresight, support, and encouragement in exploring new fields of research.

Petra Procházková wishes to thank Martin Bilej and Radka Roubalová for critical reading of the manuscript, and gratefully acknowledges support by the Ministry of Education, Youth and Sports (CZ.1.07/2.3.00/20.0055), and the Institutional Research Concepts RVO 61388971 and RVO 60077344.

CONTRIBUTORS

Diana Boraschi
CNR, Institute of Protein Biochemistry, Napoli, Italy

Laura Canesi
DISTAV, Department of Earth, Environmental and Life Sciences, University of
Genoa, Genoa, Italy

Albert Duschl
Department of Molecular Biology, University of Salzburg, Salzburg, Austria

Z. Shadi Farhangrazi
Biotrends International, Denver Technology Center, Greenwood Village, CO, USA

S. Moein Moghimi
Nanomedicine Research Group, Centre for Pharmaceutical Nanotechnology and
Nanotoxicology, University of Copenhagen; Denmark and NanoScience Centre,
University of Copenhagen, Copenhagen, Denmark

Petra Procházková
Institute of Microbiology of the Academy of Sciences of the Czech Republic,
Prague 4, Czech Republic

CHAPTER 1

How Innate and Adaptive Immunity Work

Diana Boraschi
CNR, Institute of Protein Biochemistry, Napoli, Italy

1.1 THE IMMUNE SYSTEM: PROTECTING THE BODY FROM DAMAGE

The human body exists in a hostile environment. Besides macroscopic dangers, the body needs to defend its integrity from the invisible attacks by infectious agents (bacteria, viruses, unicellular and multicellular parasites), poisons, and contaminants in air, water, and food. Other dangers come from within, those posed by the senescence, damage, or anomalous behavior of the body's own cells and tissues.

The survival and integrity of our body relies on a very sophisticated system of recognition of danger and of reaction to it, the immune system [1]. The immune system is a complex of cells and soluble factors, scattered throughout the entire body, which has the function of surveilling the body's well-being, by detecting and eliminating potentially dangerous events/agents. The immune cells patrol the body, and in particular the areas more exposed to the external environment (skin, mucosal surfaces of lung, gut, and reproductive organs). Molecules or agents that pass the mechanical barriers (mucus, keratinized epithelium, mucosa) are sampled by immune cells, which decide whether the foreign element may represent a danger or not, and act consequently. If the nonself element is considered to be a threat, the immune system mounts a defensive reaction to destroy the agents that are considered as potentially dangerous.

Which are the optimal characteristics of an effective immune response? Two are particularly important:

1. *Rapidity*: The immune reaction must be fast, leaving no time to the dangerous agent to multiply and gain access to the inner body and cause serious damage.

2. *Specificity*: The immune system must be able to discriminate between what is dangerous and what is not, so as to target the dangerous agent only and spare the surrounding cells and tissues.

How can the immune system reach the opposing goals of being both rapid and specific? In fact, being quick means having no time for developing sophisticated specific weapons, it is like firing cannonballs, which may well destroy the target but also cause substantial collateral damage. On the other hand, being specific means that some time is required for designing and building the right tools, but the risk is that during this time the dangerous agent may further invade the organism and endanger its survival.

This is why, in higher vertebrates including man, **two immune systems are active in parallel**. The innate immune system is the more primitive, rapid, and nonspecific system, with prebuilt weapons always ready to be fired. The adaptive immune system on the other hand is the sophisticated and highly specific system that, each time a dangerous agent comes in, builds new weapons specifically targeting that agent. The adaptive immune system has an additional characteristic, it can learn. This means that after having encountered a foreign agent and having designed and built the specific weapons, the cells of the system keep memory of what they have done and, if the same agent is encountered again (for instance an infective virus), the system can rebuild the specific weapons much faster and get rid of the infection much quicker.

The innate immune system is the defensive system that is already present in plants and lower animals (insects, worms, sponges, etc.). Adaptive immunity developed as consequence of a single molecular event in bony fish and, due to its evolutionary advantage for larger and long-lived species, it has been maintained and expanded into highly sophisticated system in higher vertebrates. Thus, man possesses both immune systems acting in concert. Table 1.1 summarizes the main characteristics of innate and adaptive immunity.

1.2 INNATE IMMUNITY

The innate immune system (see Chapter 2 for full details) is the more primitive defense system and is based primarily on phagocytosis [1]. Foreign agents and particles, as well as damaged cells of the own organism, are ingested and degraded by specialized cells (phagocytes). In man there are two types of phagocytes, the polymorphonuclear leukocytes (PMN or neutrophils) and the mononuclear phagocytes (monocytes/macrophages) (Table 1.2). Macrophages are scattered in all organs and tissues in the body and are the resident sentinels. When

Table 1.1 Innate Immunity Versus Adaptive Immunity

CHARACTERISTICS/FUNCTIONS	INNATE IMMUNITY	ADAPTIVE IMMUNITY
Specificity inherited in the genome	YES	NO
Receptors identical in different persons	YES	NO
Receptors present in all cells of the same type (e.g., macrophages)	YES	NO
Immediate response	YES	NO
Recognition of broad classes of molecules/agents	YES	NO
Specificity encoded in multiple gene segments	NO	YES
Requires gene rearrangement	NO	YES
Clonal distribution	NO	YES
Memory about past infection events	NO	YES
Discrimination between closely related molecular structures	NO	YES

Table 1.2 Major Immune Cells

NAME	LOCATION AND FUNCTION	IMAGE
Neutrophil granulocytes PMN	In blood, extravasate in large number within minutes and enter the inflamed tissues for destroying invading agents, phagocytic activity, produce reactive oxygen species (ROS), release granules containing proteases and antimicrobial peptides, "neutrophil extracellular traps." Short lived (about 5 days in blood, about 1−2 days in inflamed sites).	
Mononuclear phagocytes Monocytes Macrophages	Macrophages are resident in all body tissues, blood monocytes extravasate to the inflamed tissue after the PNM influx. Powerful phagocytes, release ROS, nitric oxide (NO), proteases, and inflammatory cytokines, scavengers, can present the antigen and initiate adaptive immunity. Long lived (several months).	*Three white blood cells in normal human blood: a neutrophil (lower left), a lymphocyte (middle) and a monocyte (upper right), among red blood cells.*
Lymphocytes	Circulating in the blood, located in lymphoid organs (lymph nodes, spleen, thymus). T and B lymphocytes have different functions upon activation. T cells become Th, Tc, Treg, memory T, etc. B cells mature into plasma cells that are able to produce antibodies.	

a stressful event occurs, resident macrophages detect the signals (foreign objects, extracellular matrix fragments from the damaged tissue, molecules that signal a danger released from necrotic cells, misfolded or fragmented proteins, etc.), and if these are serious they intervene directly and also call for help. The reaction of resident macrophages includes the release of alarm signals (including small proteins called chemokines) that attract other immune cells from blood to the site. The first cells that arrive are the PMN, good phagocytes, excellent in trapping and killing bacteria. PMN are short lived and precede the second wave of phagocytes, which are the blood monocytes. Monocytes are the mononuclear phagocytes of blood, similar to macrophages, they reach the site where they are activated by the same signals that have activated the resident macrophages and develop a potent killing capacity and strong phagocytic activity that contribute to the effective elimination of the foreign objects. These cells also produce cytokines, the "hormones" of the immune system, which signal to other immune cells the presence of a dangerous situation in a cascade of events that amplify the reaction until the danger is successfully eliminated. Besides phagocytes, other cells of the innate immune system are the NK cells (NK stands for natural killer), particularly important in antitumor surveillance and potent producers of IFN-γ, an inflammatory cytokine of major importance in the amplification of innate immunity.

Phagocytes use a series of receptors/sensing molecules on their plasma membrane and in their intracellular space for sampling the surrounding tissue microenvironment and for discriminating between harmless and harmful signals. The best known are the Toll-like receptors, which take their name from an antifungal receptor in insects (the protein Toll in *Drosophila melanogaster*), the first identified member of the family.

Besides effector cells, innate immunity encompasses a series of soluble factors able to bind the foreign agents and facilitate their phagocytosis and destruction. These include the collectin family proteins (such as surfactant proteins A and B), lipid transport proteins (e.g., apolipoproteins, SAA), acute-phase proteins such as short pentraxins (CRP, SAP) and long pentraxins (PTX3), and complement components, in particular C1q [1].

An important characteristic of innate immunity, which distinguishes it from adaptive immunity, is the broad recognition capacity. In fact, both the innate receptors and the innate soluble factors recognize and bind molecular patterns, that is, molecular signatures that are present in a range of different molecules. For this reason innate receptors/factors are called "pattern-recognition receptors," in contrast to receptors/antibodies that specifically recognize a single antigenic epitope.

1.3 ADAPTIVE IMMUNITY

As mentioned above, adaptive immunity is a highly sophisticated and highly specific system of recognition and response to an individual antigen (see Chapter 3) [1]. In immunology, antigen is the term that defines an entity that is specifically recognized by an antibody or a T cell receptor. Adaptive immunity coexists with innate immunity and in fact its activation depends on the preceding innate immune activity. Adaptive immunity comes into play only when innate immunity is not sufficient for solving the problem. In the case of an infection, for instance, if the infectious agent succeeds in overcoming the body barriers despite the defensive activity of innate immunity, the same innate immune cells initiate the activation of the sophisticated adaptive defense. Phagocytes that take up and degrade the invading agents are also able to "present" antigen fragments to lymphocytes, the beginning of adaptive immunity. A specialized cell population, the dendritic cells (DCs), reside in the tissues side by side with macrophages and likewise take up and digest the foreign agents. At variance with macrophages, however, once loaded DC leave the tissue and go to lymph nodes, the lymphatic stations where naïve lymphocytes reside. In the lymph node, DCs display on their surface the fragments of the invader they have digested and present them to naïve T lymphocytes. T lymphocytes have on their surface a receptor for antigens, the T cell receptor, plus a wide array of coreceptors. When the individual T lymphocyte with the right T cell receptor (i.e., one that is able to bind the antigen displayed by DC) meets the antigen-presenting DC and binds the displayed antigen, the other coreceptors stabilize the binding between DC and T cell and trigger T cell activation and proliferation, thereby hugely amplifying the number of available antigen-specific T cells. The T cell receptors, as well as B cell receptors and antibodies, can each recognize a single antigenic epitope and are able to discriminate even between very similar structures. This diversity and specificity of recognition is generated by gene rearrangement, and each lymphocyte has its own T or B cell receptor with its individual specificity, at variance with innate receptors that are germ-line encoded, have broad capacity of recognition, and are the same on all cells expressing them. Depending on the type of antigen, the activated T cells can display specific cytotoxic activity (e.g., when killing of virus-infected cells is required) or specific "helper" activity (e.g., when B lymphocytes need to be helped to produce antigen-specific antibodies). The production of antibodies, soluble molecules that specifically bind antigens and facilitate their elimination (by promoting phagocytosis, inducing complement-mediated lysis, or allowing cell-mediated killing), is performed by B lymphocytes, which upon activation become antibody-producing plasma cells, and in most cases need T cell help. T cell help is particularly important in the so-called "secondary" response, that is, the immune activation after a second challenge with the same antigen. In fact, during the first encounter with the antigen, T lymphocytes not only develop into specific effector Tc and Th cells, but also in small numbers into memory T cells, which remain quiescent until the antigen comes again. Thus, in a secondary antibody response, memory T cells remember the first encounter with the antigen and get readily activated, so that they can quickly provide help to B cells. Typically, a secondary response is much quicker than a primary response and encompasses antibodies that have undergone class switching (going from less mature IgM antibodies to IgG or IgA or IgE) and affinity maturation (higher affinity and therefore stronger binding to the antigen). There are antigens that do not trigger a T cell-dependent response, in particular polysaccharides or lipids, or antigens with repeated molecular/structural motifs. In contrast, proteins are excellent immunogens (immunogen being an antigen that can elicit a specific immune response). Thus, T cell-dependent antigens elicit an exclusively IgM response and do not induce memory, and upon second challenge develop a response similar to the first one, a type of response more similar to innate immunity rather than to an adaptive response. In contrast, T cell-dependent antigens can induce memory and, upon challenge, a much better response in terms of recognition and elimination of the antigen. This is the principle of vaccination: to induce memory against an infectious agent using protein components of the microorganism, so that, in the case of infection, the immune system is ready to mount a highly effective and protective secondary response.

1.4 NANOPARTICLES AND THE IMMUNE SYSTEM

Particles of different size and composition (from volcanic ashes to household fire smoke, from marine aerosols to viruses and bacteria) are part of our environment since the very beginning of life on this planet. Therefore, the development of our immune system has been shaped by the interaction with particulate and nanoparticulate challenges. The response to nanoparticles (NPs) by the immune system of lower environmental species, mainly based on innate type of reactions, is an important aspect of nano-ecotoxicology (see Chapter 7). The new challenge represented by engineered NPs does not differ substantially from what the immune system is used to face, although novel toxicity may result from unprecedented combinations of shape, size, charge, and chemical composition, to which the immune system has not yet adapted. In the case of nanomedicines, particles are engineered in such a way as to break barriers and to avoid immune recognition, in order to persist in the body and to deliver their drug cargo to the right site. This may be dangerous, since particles that remain in the body and are not controlled, in particular when loaded with cytotoxic drugs, may cause damage. However, escaping immune surveillance is particularly difficult, even for nanomedicines (see Chapter 6). This is indeed a long-known notion, that is, deceiving the immune system is not easy. Actually, infective viruses and bacteria have evolved through the ages by devising a number of tricks for cheating immunity, while the immune system counteracts by building additional weapons. For instance, some viruses have a gene encoding an interferon-binding protein, which can bind and therefore eliminate this major antiviral molecule produced by our cells. In some bacteria, the majority of the genome is dedicated to inhibitors of the complement system (see Chapter 2). Still, the cases in which the invader succeeds in overcoming the immune defenses are rare and, in most instances, due to weaker or anomalous functioning of the immune system, as in the case of babies (who have an immature immune system), elderly people (in which the immune system is senescent), immunosuppressive conditions (diseases, HIV infection, treatment with drugs), allergy, and autoimmunity (see Chapters 4 and 5). In these conditions of immune frailty, otherwise harmless external agents may become a problem. Thus, when assessing the safety of engineered NPs, particular attention should be devoted to the population groups at risk, that is, those immunologically frail (see Chapter 5).

REFERENCE

[1] Murphy KM. Janeway's immunobiology, eighth edition. New York, NY: Garland Science; 2011.

CHAPTER 2

Nanoparticles and Innate Immunity

Diana Boraschi

CNR, Institute of Protein Biochemistry, Napoli, Italy

2.1 THE INNATE IMMUNE SYSTEM

The innate immune system is the evolutionarily ancient defensive system that humans share with all living organisms, from plants to insects and worms, with little variation [1]. Innate immunity is based on detection of anomalous and foreign agents and molecules coming in contact with the body ("sampling" the environment), decision about the possible danger, and consequent reaction. Innate immunity has two roles: that of maintaining the integrity of function of the body, by detecting and eliminating senescent or damaged cells, proteins, and other molecules; and that of immediate defense against foreign invading agents. Thus, innate immunity probes its microenvironment and interacts with all the elements present. If the interacting element is considered harmless, the innate immune system does not react. If, on the other hand, it is felt as potentially dangerous, a defensive reaction ensues.

Innate immunity and inflammation are in many instances used as synonyms, to describe the rapid nonspecific defensive reaction to invaders. Inflammation is a complex series of events, starting with the innate immune system detecting and reacting to stressful agents or events, and developing with recruitment of other cells and, in many instances, of adaptive immunity, in order to eliminate the danger. There are two major types of inflammation. Type 1 inflammation is a reaction aiming at killing bacteria and other microorganisms, or at killing the body's own cells if they have been virally infected or become tumor cells. In this response, the inflammatory cytokines IL-12, IL-18, and IFN-γ are abundantly produced and activate T_H1-mediated adaptive immunity. Conversely, type 2 inflammation is the reaction triggered by multicellular parasites (such as worms), in which IL-4 is the major cytokine and T_H2-dependent adaptive immunity is activated. Both types of response are activated for destroying dangerous agents, and both resolve with shutting off the immune response when it is no longer needed, and with the repair of the damages to the tissue caused by the reaction itself. Throughout this book they will be referred to as type 1 and type 2 adaptive immune response, to prevent confusion with the innate immunity that is also sometimes described by the term "inflammation."

It should be underlined that, as innate immunity is the first, fast-acting defensive system of the body, its goal is that of keeping off potential dangers by any possible means. If they cannot be eradicated, they have at least to be locally contained (resulting in local inflammation), while the body is busy building a specific strategy (adaptive immunity). The consequence is that **rapidity equals lack of specificity**, as there is no time for an accurate choice of targets. Thus, privileging rapidity causes a certain number of mistakes, in particular when foreign molecules are similar to those displayed by our own cells, with the risk of autoreactivity that is at the basis of autoimmune syndromes.

As mentioned in Chapter 1, the innate immune system encompasses a series of effector cells and an array of soluble factors. The major characteristic of innate immunity is that the genes coding for its sensing receptors and structures and for its factors are germ line encoded, which means that they are always the same, without rearrangements or changes ever occurring. There is no *bona fide* immunological memory in innate immunity, and its activity is fully efficient at the first encounter with an invader and it will still be the same after repeated encounters (see Table 1.1 in Chapter 1 for the differences between innate and adaptive immunity).

2.2 THE INNATE IMMUNE CELLS

Innate immune effector cells are leukocytes residing in the blood and, upon extravasation, scattered throughout the entire body [1]. Leukocytes that enter a tissue do it either as a physiological homeostatic mechanism, that is, for replenishing the pool of resident sentinel cells, or during the course of an inflammatory reaction in the tissues, for helping the resident sentinels to combat the danger. Innate leukocytes include monocytes (about 5% of white blood cells (WBC) and their mature tissue-residing counterpart, macrophages) and polymorphonuclear leukocytes that encompass neutrophils (PMN; about 60% of WBC). Less frequent are eosinophils (about 2% of WBC, important for responses to parasites), and basophils (0.4% of WBC, also involved in antiparasite activity), as well as **dendritic cells** (DCs) and innate lymphoid cells (ILCs; [2]) of which the best characterized are natural killer (NK) cells (Table 2.1).

Resident innate immune cells are mainly **tissue macrophages**, highly differentiated phagocytic cells derived from blood monocytes that have the primary role of scavengers that are patrolling the tissue and eating and eliminating all debris (including the body's own dying and anomalous cells) and invading external agents. Tissue macrophages are different in each tissue, as they adapt to the different microenvironment and required functions: alveolar macrophages in the lung; osteoclasts in the bone; Kupffer cells in the liver; microglial cells in the brain; Langerhans cells in the skin; and histiocytes, interdigitating cells, and veiled cells in connective and other tissues [1,3].

Other cells that are similar to macrophages are the DCs, less efficient in phagocytosis and more efficient in antigen presentation as compared to macrophages. DCs, for their ability to present antigens to T cells, may be considered the first responding cells of adaptive immunity, and therefore will be addressed in Chapter 3.

Another important leukocyte is the **neutrophil** or PMN, the most abundant type in WBC [1,4]. PMNs are the very first cells that intervene in a tissue after an insult, and their destructive activity is fast and powerful, with degranulation and release of proteases, oxidizing enzymes, ROS, and a series of other toxic compounds (for killing microorganisms), with phagocytosis, and by releasing the neutrophil extracellular traps (NETs), which are true nets of DNA filaments decorated with granules filled with enzymes and toxic peptides [5].

NK cells are a type of innate lymphocytes, present both in the blood and scattered in tissues. NK cells have a receptor system that allows them to distinguish between normal cells and anomalous cells, and a lytic machinery that they use for killing such cells. NK cells are half way between innate and adaptive cells, as they seem to be capable of some form of memory, like T cells and unlike innate leukocytes [1,6].

2.3 SENSING OF NANOPARTICLES BY INNATE IMMUNE CELLS

Innate effector cells can probe the surrounding microenvironment with an array of sensing molecules. These innate receptors recognize

Table 2.1 Innate Immune Effector Cells

NAME	PERCENT IN WBC	DIAMETER (μm)	LIFESPAN	CHARACTERISTICS	FUNCTION	MICROSCOPIC IMAGE
Monocyte	5%	15–20	Few days	Kidney-shaped nucleus	Exits the blood stream for replenishing the macrophage tissue pools and in the case of inflammatory events (different subpopulations)	
Macrophage	Exclusively in tissues	20–60	Months to years	Large cytoplasm, dendrites, can form multinucleated giant cells	Phagocytic scavenger in tissues, derived from monocytes, can present antigen, sentinel against pathogens, produce toxic ROS and NO	
Dendritic cell	0.4%, in most tissues	15–20	Months to years in tissues	Long dendrites	Derived from monocytes or from B cells, in tissues can pick up antigen and migrate to lymph nodes, where they present antigen to T cells	
Neutrophil	60%	12–15	Hours	Multilobed nucleus, neutrophilic cytoplasm with HE staining	Defense against pathogens and foreign agents through phagocytosis, degranulation, ROS, and NETs	
Eosinophil	2%	12–15	10 days (hours in circulation)	Bilobed nucleus, pink granules with HE staining	Effector cell in parasite infections, also involved in allergies	

Basophil	0.4%	12–15	Hours to days	Bi- or trilobed nucleus, dark blue granules with HE staining	Inflammatory cell, releases histamine upon IgE binding	
Mast cell	Exclusively in tissues	15–20	Months to years	Round nucleus, dark blue granules with HE staining	Functions similar to basophils, but origin is different	
NK	3%, in tissues	10–15	Few days	Large granular lymphocytes	Antitumor surveillance, strong cytolytic activity	

molecular patterns rather than specific molecular sequences/structures, and are therefore called "pattern-recognition receptors" (PRRs). The patterns recognized by PRRs are molecular signatures shared by different molecules or agents, having in common the fact that they are displayed by pathogenic microorganisms or are in any case different from the body's own molecular patterns. These molecular signatures are generally called "pathogen-associated molecular patterns" (PAMPs). Just to give an example, the innate receptor TLR4 recognizes an array of PAMPs from bacteria (Gram-negative lipopolysaccharide—also known as LPS or endotoxin, heat shock proteins (HSPs)), viruses (Rous Sarcoma Virus (RSV) protein F, Vesicular Stomatitis Virus (VSV) glycoprotein G), fungi (molecules from *Candida albicans*, *Aspergillus fumigatus* conidia and hyphae, *C. neoformans* capsular polysaccharides, mannan), and multicellular parasites (*Trypanosoma* glycoinositolphospholipids).

Toll-like receptors (TLRs) are a group of PRRs that take their name from the antifungal *Drosophila* receptor Toll. In man, there are 10 TLRs (TLR1−10) that can form hetero- or homodimers/multimers and have recognition capacity for large arrays of PAMPs [1,7]. Some TLRs are expressed on the plasma membrane of cells, being effective in detecting extracellular PAMPs. On the other hand, TLRs involved in detection of viral components are present intracellularly, displayed on the membrane of intracellular vesicles (Table 2.2). TLRs are expressed by many cell types, but they represent the major pathogen-sensing tool and activation receptor of mononuclear phagocytes, which in fact display a full array of coreceptors and transporters that allow correct TLR activation.

The possibility that nanoparticles (NPs) may directly interact with TLRs, thereby activating the innate/inflammatory defensive system, has been investigated by several groups, who found that different NPs are inflammatory through interaction with and activation of TLRs (see, e.g., Ref. [8]). All these results are however to be considered in light of the possible contamination of the NPs used in experimental systems with one or more of the *bona fide* TLR ligands, which are ubiquitous in our normal environment. As in the case of the alleged endogenous TLR ligands (see Section 2.5), no formal proof has been yet obtained that TLR binding and activation by NPs occurs directly and is not mediated by the presence of trace amounts (often hard to detect) of LPS, lipopeptides, or other microbial-derived molecules. On

Table 2.2 TLRs in Human Leukocytes[a]

RECEPTOR	LOCATION	CELLS	LIGANDS	LIGAND ORIGIN
TLR1	Plasma membrane	Monocytes, macrophages, immature myeloid DC, neutrophils, eosinophils, mast cells, NK, B cells	Triacyl lipopeptides	Bacteria
TLR2	Plasma membrane	Monocytes, macrophages, myeloid DC, neutrophils, eosinophils, basophils, mast cells, NK, B cells (low), T cells	Glycolipids, lipopeptides, lipoproteins	Bacteria, parasites
			Lipoteichoic acid	Gram-positive bacteria
			Zymosan	Fungi
			HSP70 (?)	Host
			HSV, VSV, CMV	Viruses
			Others	
TLR3	Intracellular	Mature myeloid DC, mast cells, NK, B cells	dsRNA, PolyI:C	Viruses
TLR4	Plasma membrane and intracellular	Monocytes, macrophages, myeloid DC, neutrophils, eosinophils, basophils, mast cells, NK, B cells (low)	Lipopolysaccharide, lipid A	Gram-negative bacteria
			HSP	Bacteria, host (?)
			Structural proteins	Viruses
			Mannan	Fungi
			Fragments of fibrinogen, hyaluronate, heparan sulfate (?)	Host
			GPIL	Trypanosome
TLR5	Plasma membrane	Monocytes, macrophages, myeloid DC, neutrophils, eosinophils, NK cells	Flagellin	Bacteria
TLR6	Plasma membrane	Monocytes, macrophages, myeloid DC, neutrophils, eosinophils, mast cells, NK, B cells	Diacyl lipopeptides	Bacteria
TLR7	Intracellular	Monocytes, macrophages, plasmacytoid DC, neutrophils, eosinophils, mast cells (lung), B cells (low)	ssRNA (imidazoquinoline and analogues)	RNA viruses
TLR8	Intracellular	Monocytes, macrophages, myeloid DC, neutrophils, mast cells, NK	ssRNA (imidazoquinoline and analogues)	RNA viruses
TLR9	Intracellular	Monocytes, macrophages, plasmacytoid DC, neutrophils, eosinophils, mast cells (skin), NK, B cells	Unmethylated CpG DNA	Bacteria, DNA viruses

(Continued)

Table 2.2 (Continued)				
RECEPTOR	**LOCATION**	**CELLS**	**LIGANDS**	**LIGAND ORIGIN**
TLR10	Plasma membrane	Monocytes, macrophages, DC, neutrophils, eosinophils, mast cells (lung), NK, B cells	Unknown	Unknown

[a]Heteroassociation of TLR2 with TLR1, TLR6, and TLR10 has been shown. In the mouse, TLR11−13 have been described, while TLR10 is missing.

the other hand, NP modification with TLR ligands is one of the most promising directions in the design of immunostimulating vaccine adjuvants (see Chapter 6).

Other innate PRRs are the C-type lectin receptors (CLRs, including Dectin-1 and DC-SIGN), and scavenger receptors (SR-A and SR-B), expressed on the phagocyte plasma membrane, and different classes of intracytoplasmic receptor families such as the NOD-like receptors (NLRs) and the RIG-I-like receptors (Table 2.2). The NP surface coating (for instance with carbohydrates such as dextran) facilitates recognition by certain classes of innate receptors and uptake by macrophages [9]. This would suggest that interaction with innate cells may occur through different receptors and with different modalities not only as a consequence of engineered surface modification but also following unintentional surface decoration (e.g., with molecules adsorbed from the microenvironment and from surrounding bacteria). NPs that gain access to the cytoplasm may interact with NLRs, a family of proteins that can sense intracytoplasmic danger signals and initiate the assembly of a protein complex called "inflammasome," leading to the activation of the enzyme caspase-1 and the consequent maturation and release of the inflammatory cytokines IL-1β and IL-18 [10]. The classical macrophage inflammasome based on the NLR protein NLRP3 can sense a wide array of signals (K^+ efflux induced by a variety of agents including ATP and TLR stimulation, bacteria such as *Staphylococcus aureus* and *Listeria monocytogenes*, bacterial RNA, and uric acid crystals). It has been reported, although the evidence is debated, that the most used vaccine adjuvant alum (particles of aluminum hydroxide on which the immunogen is adsorbed) can amplify the immune response because it induces inflammasome activation and production of the inflammatory and immunostimulatory cytokine IL-1β [11]. The hypothesis that NPs can activate the inflammasome has led to a huge effort in nanomedicine in functionalizing the NP surface to gain access to NLRP3 within macrophages and DCs, in order to achieve not only the delivery of the immunogen to the antigen-presenting cells but also the stimulation of innate immunity that is required to obtain effective immunization [12]. The other side of the story is that, as in the case of uric acid crystals in gout, the persistence of inflammasome activation and IL-1β production is the basis of chronic inflammatory diseases (see Section 2.6).

2.4 INTERACTION OF NANOPARTICLES WITH INNATE IMMUNE CELLS

Interaction of NPs with monocytes and macrophages has been widely studied in a range of cellular models *in vitro* and also *in vivo* in experimental animals. *In vivo*, the overall observation (obtained in pharmacokinetics experiments for nanomedicine) is that, in particular for metal NPs, particles that are not readily excreted are significantly taken up by the mononuclear phagocyte system in particular in spleen, liver, and lung [13]. Interaction with mononuclear phagocytes depends heavily on the route of entry into the body and on the consequent **"coating" of the reactive NP surface with microenvironmental proteins**, for instance surfactant proteins for inhaled particles coming in contact with alveolar macrophages, or serum albumin for NPs administered intravenously and coming in contact with circulating monocytes [14]. This means that our innate cells do in fact come in contact not directly with the NPs, but rather with the molecules that are decorating their surface, the same that happens when encountering bacteria or foreign bodies. Indeed, the adsorption of "self" molecules ("self" meaning intrinsic to the body, as opposed to "nonself") on the surface is one of the ways for the immune system to combat invasion. Recognition and destruction is facilitated if the foreign agent is "opsonized", that is, covered with antibodies or complement components (see Section 2.5 for definition of complement), while innate immunity is set on alarm if the foreign surface modifies the structure of self molecules like hyaluronic acid or fibrinogen [1,15]. On the other hand, getting covered with the body's molecules is one of the successful strategies that pathogens use for escaping innate recognition (see for instance the capacity of *Neisseria meningitidis* of covering its surface with the host's factor H, which is a potent inhibitor of the lytic activity of complement) [16]. Therefore, the ability of NPs to adsorb different types of molecules in a particular tissue microenvironment may make a huge difference in the capacity of innate immunity to recognize them as foreign entities and to mount an inflammatory response. Thus, the great body of experimental studies accumulated in the past years may need to be reassessed in light of the validity of the systems used in representing the real-life situation, even for the data obtained with human normal cells. Naked NPs were often directly added to the culture medium usually containing fetal calf serum (circumstances that hardly reproduce what may happen to human beings in real life), or used on macrophage-like tumor cell lines (transformed cells that may not reproduce the behavior of normal cells), or tested in animals or on animal cells (which may not always reflect the human reactivity) [17]. It has to be shown that the various models systems mirror the human reactions *in vivo*, before we can accept them as representing the impact of NPs on human cells. The great variability of results in the literature may in part depend on the artificial and poorly representative systems often used [18].

In general, given their role as scavengers, **macrophages tend to take up foreign particles**, including NPs covered with altered self proteins, and they do it by using different mechanisms depending on the particle size and surface coating [19]. Aggregation of particles, which occurs in several instances in contact with biological fluids, increases the particle size and facilitates phagocytosis. "Opsonization" with complement components or immunoglobulins also facilitates particle uptake by receptor-mediated endocytosis. When particles are too big or fiber-like (in the case of NPs, this occurs only in the case of rigid nanotubes), macrophages fail to engulf them and may die while trying, an event that in the 1980s was designated with the name of "frustrated phagocytosis." On the other hand, macrophages can fuse and form multinucleated giant cells or syncitia that surround and seclude the foreign body. The inability to get rid of the foreign agent leads to a local persistent inflammation that in many cases causes a fibrotic reaction (in which macrophages play a major role) that firmly encapsulates the undigestible foreign agent, to avoid its coming in contact with the body's inner tissues [1]. In a few cases, a severe pathology may ensue (as in the case of inhaled asbestos fibers, which can cause mesothelioma, a pleural tumor) [20,21].

PMNs can interact with NPs similarly to what they do with bacteria, thus they can take them up, trap them with NETs, and attack them extracellularly with enzymes and oxidizing compounds. In the case of carbon-based NPs (e.g., single- and multiwalled carbon nanotubes, graphene), it has been observed that myeloperoxidase, an oxidative enzyme abundantly produced by neutrophils and also by eosinophils and macrophages, can effectively degrade the nanotubes that, once degraded, lose their ability to cause lung inflammation when inhaled by mice [22,23]. PMNs can also use NETs for entrapping and concentrating NPs into some sort of granulomas that bar them from coming in contact with the body's tissues [24].

Regarding NK cells, while there is abundant literature on the capacity of NPs delivered *in vivo* to enhance NK recruitment and activity (which is part of an ongoing innate reaction to a stressful event), no solid evidence exists of a direct interaction. Also in this case, surface modification of NPs is being attempted for building nanomedicines able to enhance NK activity in tumors or for carrying drugs to the tumor site through recruited NK cells.

2.5 INTERACTION WITH INNATE IMMUNE FACTORS

Soluble factors of innate immunity encompass several classes of molecules that are active in binding PAMPs and facilitate their destruction (Table 2.3).

A very efficient soluble system of pathogen recognition and destruction is **complement** [1]. The complement system is composed by a series of proteins and enzymes that activate each other in a cascade, generating a series of bioactive intermediates, and ending up with the formation of a "hole" in the membrane of bacteria (Table 2.4). The complement cascade is initiated through three different pathways. The classical pathway is activated by the C1 complex, starting with C1q binding to an antibody complexed to an antigen, or directly binding to the surface of a pathogen. The alternative pathway is always active at low levels and attacks the surface of every cell, avoiding to kill the organism's own cells only because they possess protective factors while bacteria do not. The lectin pathway is very similar to the classical pathway but it is initiated by pathogen recognition by the mannose-binding lectin (MBL), a molecule structurally very similar to C1q, which recognizes the specific spacing of mannose residues on bacterial surfaces. Complement activation is of great efficacy in eliminating infectious microorganisms, not only by direct killing but also by

Table 2.3 The Major Soluble Innate Immunity Factors in Man

FACTOR	CHARACTERISTICS	TARGET	FUNCTION	
			PHYSIOLOGICAL	DEFENSIVE
Pentraxins				
CRP	Small pentraxin, annular pentamer, acute phase protein (produced by liver)	Phosphocholine on dying cell surface or on microbial surfaces	Detection and elimination of dying cells, avoids recognition by DC	Opsonization, facilitates complement binding
Serum amyloid P component (SAP)	Negatively charged carbohydrates		Unknown	Opsonization, facilitates complement binding
PTX3 (TSG-14)	Long pentraxin, produced by leukocytes and other cells	C1q, apoptotic cells, microorganisms, TNFAIP6	Detection and elimination of dying cells, avoids recognition by DC	Microbial opsonization, activates classical complement pathway
Ficolins (Fibrinogen- and collagen-containing lectins)				
M-ficolin (Ficolin-1)	Produced by leukocytes	N-acetylglucosamine, sialic acid	Binds to PTX3 and together promote elimination of dying cells	Binds to all bacteria with surface sialic acid (e.g. Streptococcus), activating complement
L-ficolin (Ficolin-2)	Produced in liver, pattern-recognition molecule	Acetylated sugars, certain 1,3-β-glucans	Unknown	Activates the lectin pathway of complement, cooperates with PTX3 and collectins in microbial elimination
H-ficolin (Ficolin-3)	Abundant in serum is associated with MASP	Acetylated sugars, bacteria, viruses	Unknown	Binds several viruses and promotes activation of complement
Collectins (collagen-containing C-type lectins)				
MBL	Polymeric, at least a tetramer is needed for complement activation	Carbohydrate patterns on a variety of microorganisms	Binds apoptotic and senescent cells, promoting their elimination	Binds to bacteria, viruses, protozoa, fungi, and starts the lectin pathway of complement activation
SP-A and SP-D (surfactant proteins A and D)	In lung alveoli	Carbohydrates on fungi and bacteria, SP-A can directly bind LPS	Regulates secretion of pulmonary surfactant	Opsonization of microorganisms, promoting their interaction with lung effector leukocytes

Lipid transport proteins

Apolipoproteins	Synthesized in intestine and liver, many different types	Lipids, to form lipoproteins; bacterial LPS	Transport of lipids and regulation of lipid metabolism	Neutralization of LPS and bacterial clearance
sCD14	Soluble form of the CD14 coreceptor for LPS, expressed by monocytes and macrophages	Endogenous phosphatidylinositol, phosphatidylethanolamine; bacterial LPS, phosphatidylglycerol, lipoteichoic acid	Lipid transfer	Coreceptor for LPS, shuttle of PAMPs to TLRs, in cooperation with BPI and LBP
BPI (bactericidal permeability increasing protein)	Produced by neutrophils and other cells, endogenous antibiotic	Phosphatidylcholine, LPS	Lipid transfer	Binds and neutralizes LPS, cooperates with LBP in activating innate immunity
LBP (lipopolysaccharide-binding protein)	Produced by macrophages and other cells	Phosphatidylinositol, phosphatidylcholine and phosphatidylethanolamine; lipid A of LPS	Lipid transfer	Shuttle of PAMPs to TLRs, in cooperation with BPI, CD14
CETP (colesteryl ester transfer protein)	Plasma protein	Colesteryl ester, triglycerides	Lipid transfer between lipoproteins	Unknown
PLTP (phospholipid transfer protein)	Plasma protein	Phospholipids, LPS	Phospholipid transfer between lipoproteins	Neutralization of LPS and bacterial clearance
PLUNC (palate, lung and nasal epithelium carcinoma associated protein)	Secreted in neutrophil granules, expressed in upper airways, up-regulated in inflammation	Highly hydrophobic	Lung surfactant	Inhibits bacterial biofilms

Alarmins

HSPs	Includes many molecules, found in many living organisms, including bacteria	LPS, proteins	Intracellular protein chaperones, facilitate antigen uptake and presentation, in particular for viral antigens	DAMPs, facilitate LPS binding to TLR4

(Continued)

Table 2.3 (Continued)				
			FUNCTION	
FACTOR	CHARACTERISTICS	TARGET	PHYSIOLOGICAL	DEFENSIVE
High-mobility group box 1 (HMGB1)	Nuclear factor, released by macrophages during inflammation	LPS, RAGE (receptor)	Transcription factors	Shuttle of LPS to sCD14, when released actively or by dying cells is chemotactic for leukocytes and has proliferative and angiogenic capacity
Fragments of matrix components	Fragments of hyaluronate, fibronectin, heparan sulfate released in damaged matrix	May bind LPS and other bacterial lipid-containing components	Stimulate tissue reconstruction	DAMPs, induce inflammatory activation of phagocytes
S100 proteins	Produced by macrophages and DC	Heparan sulfate, proteoglycans, carboxylated N-glycans, Ca^{++}-binding protein	Phosphorylation, homeostatic regulation of cytoskeleton, and other intracellular functions	When released extracellularly, inflammatory activation of leukocytes and endothelial cells
IL-1α	Member of the IL-1 family, cell-associated and soluble forms (released upon cell death)	IL-1 receptors	Intracellular form is a transcription factor	Released form has inflammatory activity, similar to IL-1β
Galectins	β-Galactoside-binding lectins, dimers to pentamers, produced by several cell types, active within and outside cells	β-Galactoside sugars (N-acetyl-lactosamines)	Regulation of apoptosis, T cell proliferation, T cell receptor functions; Gal3 inhibits macrophage inflammation	Considered as DAMPs; pathogens may use them for promoting their own survival
Cathelicidins	Cationic amphipathic peptides, in humans LL-37 and hCAP-18, found in lysosomes of neutrophils and macrophages	Lipid membranes of bacteria, within phagolysosomes	None	Strong antimicrobial activity (broad-spectrum endogenous antibiotics), chemotactic, amplifies inflammatory responses
β-Defensins	Cysteine-rich cationic proteins, produced by leukocytes	LPS, bacterial lipid membranes	None	Antimicrobial activity, chemotactic, activates TLRs (by shuttling LPS?)

Table 2.4 The Complement System

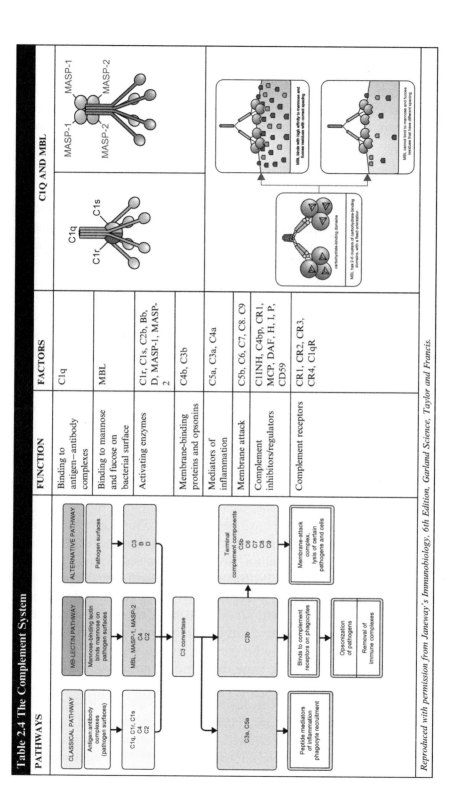

PATHWAYS	FUNCTION	FACTORS	C1Q AND MBL
	Binding to antigen–antibody complexes	C1q	
	Binding to mannose and fucose on bacterial surface	MBL	
	Activating enzymes	C1r, C1s, C2b, Bb, D, MASP-1, MASP-2	
	Membrane-binding proteins and opsonins	C4b, C3b	
	Mediators of inflammation	C5a, C3a, C4a	
	Membrane attack	C5b, C6, C7, C8, C9	
	Complement inhibitors/regulators	C1INH, C4bp, CR1, MCP, DAF, H, I, P, CD59	
	Complement receptors	CR1, CR2, CR3, CR4, C1qR	

Reproduced with permission from Janeway's Immunobiology, 6th Edition, Garland Science, Taylor and Francis.

triggering inflammation, because complement fragments have diverse activities including opsonization (i.e., they can coat the surface of foreign agents, thereby facilitating their recognition and uptake by phagocytes through complement receptors), chemotaxis for leukocytes, and triggering of their inflammatory activation. On the other hand, prolonged or systemic complement activation may cause huge damage and serious pathologies (including hemolysis).

The **capacity of NPs to activate complement** has been widely studied, as this is a significant safety issue in nanomedicine. Size, shape, surface characteristics, and also the hosts genetic polymorphisms may affect the recognition of NPs by the complement system and the initiation of an adverse reaction, and therefore this represents one of the major issues in the design of safe nanomedicines [25,26]. It is particularly interesting, in this perspective, that C1q and MBL are able to recognize not only some types of molecules but, importantly, their repetitive and spacial order. Thus, repeated and ordered molecular motifs (as they occur in many nanomaterials) can make the NP readily recognizable by complement. To avoid complement activation in nanomedicine, an important lesson can be learned by studying the complement-escaping strategies used by bacteria, which can dedicate to complement modulation a large part of their genome [27], as in the already mentioned case of *N. meningitidis* that captures the host's factor H and covers its own surface with it to avoid activating the alternative complement pathway [28].

Other soluble innate factors are pentraxins, ficolins, collectins (collagen-containing C-type lectins), and the lipid transport proteins. **Pentraxins** are pattern-recognition soluble molecules with a typical pentaradial structure [29,30]. Pentraxins include acute phase proteins such as the C-reactive protein (CRP) and PTX3, which are produced during acute inflammation, and are able to bind microbial structures favoring their uptake and destruction by promoting binding via the Fc receptors (receptors for antibodies present on the surface of phagocytes). PTX3 is also able to activate the complement classical pathway by binding to C1q. **Ficolins** are circulating proteins that recognize several molecular patterns including acylated sugars and certain β-glucans [1,31]. L-ficolin is one of the molecules that can activate the complement lectin pathway, similar to MBL [32]. **Collectins** are a group of proteins that include the already mentioned MBL (that activates the lectin pathway of complement), and surfactant proteins A and D. Collectins bind to sugars or lipids on the microbial surface and facilitate their recognition and elimination. Thus, collectins can promote microbial aggregation and act as opsonins, thereby facilitating phagocytosis and activating complement (see MBL) [31]. **Lipid-binding proteins** have the role of transporting lipids within the body, and include apolipoproteins, sCD14, BPI, LBP, CETP, PLTP, and PLUNC. All these proteins have a physiological role in binding and transporting endogenous lipids, but all of them can also recognize and bind bacterial LPSs and other bacterial structures and contribute to their neutralization and elimination, being also involved in the modulation of the innate immune response.

A last group of soluble innate factors can be mentioned, that is, the alarmins. **Alarmins** are a diverse group of endogenous molecules that can set the innate immune system into alarm, and they are also known as damage-associated molecular patterns (DAMPs). They are self molecules whose presence in a particular situation is not normal, or that are produced only in anomalous situations. Thus, alarmins include HSPs or HMGB1 outside of the cells, when in normal conditions they are always inside, or fragments of matrix components such as hyaluronate, fibrinogen, and heparan sulfate (which indicate tissue damage). In addition, alarmins include a series of factors released by cells (in particular phagocytes) for starting the inflammatory reaction such as S100 proteins, IL-1α, galectins (β-galactoside-binding lectins), cathelicidins, and β-defensins [14,33]. In the past, several alarmins had been reported as being able to bind directly to innate receptors, and activate the innate/inflammatory reaction in the absence of a microbial challenge. A thorough critical analysis of the experimental data however has shed some doubt, as in several cases it was impossible to rule out the presence of trace amounts of microbial molecules (LPS and others) [34]. Thus, while direct innate activation may be more limited than initially thought, the major role of soluble innate factors remains that of facilitating innate receptor activation upon foreign pattern recognition, acting as PAMP-sensitizing molecules (transporters, coreceptors, focalizing molecules) and amplifiers of the response.

While little is known of the possible interaction between NPs and any of these innate factors, a recent report has examined the role of sPLUNC1 in the inflammatory response to single-walled carbon nanotubes (SWCNTs), showing that binding of sPLUNC1 to SWCNT could decrease their ability to stimulate inflammatory cytokine production by mouse macrophages *in vitro* [35]. It could be hypothesized that NPs covered with endogenous molecules (either innate soluble factors or self molecules that may change their structure upon interaction with the NPs surface) may actually act as alarmins [36]. In nanomedicine, conjugation of alarmins (e.g., galectin-1) on NPs is being attempted for selective targeting to receptor-expressing cells and their functional modulation [37].

2.6 INNATE IMMUNE REACTION TO NANOPARTICLES: HEALING VERSUS CHRONIC INFLAMMATION

In light of all the information given above, predicting if and how the innate immune system will react to NPs is hard. We have seen above a brief summary of some of the wide array of different tools that the innate immune system has developed for facing whatever kind of dangers will come about, tools that are **redundant** (i.e., there are different factors or cells that can do the same thing, while the same cell or factor can do different things), in order to make sure that nothing ever goes undetected. Thus, if NPs are seen as a possible danger, innate immunity will be activated and an inflammatory response will be started. This is actually good news, because it means that our defenses are efficient and know how to take care of the problems. We will see in Chapter 5 the possible risks that could derive from failing immunity in some conditions of immunological frailty.

An **innate/inflammatory reaction has its well-defined course limited in time** [1]. The reaction is triggered by the encounter between a dangerous agent and the innate immune system, and it develops with the activation of resident cells and the recruitment into the site of other effector cells (which come in waves, first the PMNs, then the monocytes and subsequently, in some cases, also the lymphocytes) that generate a complex reaction ending up with the elimination of the dangerous agent. The absence of the initial trigger, which has been destroyed, leads to a substantial change of the microenvironment that redirects the activity of the phagocytes toward tissue reconstruction (production of anti-inflammatory factors, elimination of dead cells and debris, stimulation of fibroblast proliferation and of angiogenesis, production of matrix components, etc.), to reestablish tissue homeostasis and functions. Wound healing is thus the final phase of a successful immune defense.

It is only in few special circumstances that the reaction does not follow this course, thereby causing pathological consequences. A typical case of **anomalous inflammation**, in which the inflammatory phase is eliminated, is that of solid tumors, which can create a mocking microenvironment for the incoming inflammatory macrophages that immediately directs them into noninflammatory tissue-promoting activity, thus avoiding being killed and at the same time exploiting macrophage functions for promoting tumor growth. An opposite example, in which the inflammatory phase is abnormally extended, is that of chronic inflammatory, degenerative, and autoimmune diseases. A typical example is that of infectious agents that display molecules similar or identical with the body's own components, therefore triggering a response that cannot ever stop because the recognized molecule is part of the body and will always be present. In these cases, the final phase of the inhibition of inflammation and tissue reconstruction, which is actually triggered by inflammatory signals in an autoregulatory loop, is activated and acts concomitantly to inflammation, in the impossible attempt to down-regulate it. Thus, in many of these chronic diseases we can find an anomalous mixture of exaggerated activation of both inflammatory and anti-inflammatory mechanisms, with concomitant tissue destruction and tissue neoformation (as in the case of rheumatoid arthritis), that all contribute to the pathology.

Thus, regarding the possible effects of NPs on innate immunity and inflammation, we should ask two questions:

1. **Can NPs trigger an inflammatory reaction?**
2. If yes, **does this inflammatory reaction resolve, or will it persist?**

A key issue here, in order to correctly evaluate the capacity of NPs to trigger inflammation, is the assessment of the cleanliness of the NPs under study. Contamination with bacterial fragments, even of materials that are sterile (i.e., not containing living microorganisms), is very common unless special precautions are taken. In particular, the most potent activator of inflammation, that is, **Gram-negative LPS (or endotoxin), is a ubiquitous contaminant of biomaterials** that can be eliminated only with difficulty [18,38]. Thus, to avoid examining the inflammatory effects of contaminating endotoxin, it is of utmost importance using endotoxin-free NPs in the experimental procedures *in vitro* and *in vivo* (see, for instance, Ref. [39]). Methods for testing the presence of endotoxin in NP preparations are not standardized [40] and need accurate validation before being applicable to NPs [41]. Despite these problems, accurately measuring endotoxin in NPs, thereby being able to using endotoxin-free NPs, is mandatory in order to discriminate between confounding inflammatory effects caused by the contaminant and true NP-dependent effects.

Several NPs can be degraded or can dissolve once they are in contact with biological fluids or cell. Thus, in the majority of cases, dealing with NPs is, for the innate immune system, no bigger problem than having to deal with bacteria or viruses or damaged proteins, unless the components into which the NPs are dissociating are toxic (like some metal ions). A problem may be posed by NPs that cannot be degraded and that therefore risk to remain for prolonged periods within the body. Also in this case, however, innate immunity has its strategies. Phagocytes can accumulate around the foreign body and form a barrier around it (fibrous capsules, granulomas), to separate it from the surrounding tissue and avoid dangerous interactions. In some cases, the foreign bodies can be transported through the lymph or even the circulation systems to the periphery and extruded from the organism. Thus, **cases where NPs may persist in the body** at such concentrations as to overcome all the defensive systems and to cause chronic inflammation **are exceptional**. One case is that of gout, in which micro- and nanocrystals of uric acid secreted by cells accumulate in joints, enter phagocytes, and stimulate the NLRP3 inflammasome, with consequent IL-1β production and ensuing inflammation. Inflammation persists as long as the crystals continue being formed [42]. Another case is that of asbestos fibers that can cause mesothelioma in the pleura, although the mechanisms of tumor development are far from clear, and the relationship between tumor development with fiber-induced inflammation is not established [43].

Obviously, poisonous NPs may overcome the immune system simply because they can kill cells that ingest them. This is one of the dangers of nanomedicines loaded with chemotherapeutic drugs for antitumor therapy, as a large part of these NPs is actually taken up by leukocytes, with the risk of selectively eliminating the innate immune defenses [13,19].

On the other hand, the fact that NPs can adsorb on their surface the body's self-molecules, may change the molecule (by changing its shape and its folding) in a way that makes it immunogenic, that is, recognizable by the adaptive immune system, which will then mount a specific response against it. This possibility will be addressed more in detail in Chapter 3. Suffice to say, no formal proof exists to date that this event can really occur. Nevertheless, considering this possibility is an important part of the studies for implementing NP safety.

REFERENCES

[1] Murphy KM. Janeway's immunobiology, eighth edition. New York, NY: Garland Science; 2011.

[2] Walker JA, Barlow JL, McKenzie ANJ. Innate lymphoid cells—how did we miss them? Nat Rev Immunol 2013;13:75–87.

[3] The Macrophage Community Website. <www.macrophages.com>. [Accessed September 2013].

[4] Witko-Sarsat V, Rieu P, Descamps-Latscha B, Lesavre P, Halbwachs-Mecarelli L. Neutrophils: molecules, functions and pathophysiological aspects. Lab Invest 2000;80:617–53.

[5] Papayannopoulos V, Zychlinsky A. NETs: a new strategy for using old weapons. Trends Immunol 2009;30:513–21.

[6] Sun JC, Lanier LL. Natural killer cells remember: an evolutionary bridge between innate and adaptive immunity? Eur J Immunol 2009;39:2059–64.

[7] O'Neill LAJ, Golenbock D, Bowie AG. The history of Toll-like receptors—redefining innate immunity. Nat Rev Immunol 2013;13:453–60.

[8] Mano SS, Kanehira K, Taniguchi A. Comparison of cellular uptake and inflammatory response via Toll-like receptor 4 to lipopolysaccharide and titanium dioxide nanoparticles. Int J Mol Sci 2013;14:13154–70.

[9] Chao Y, Karmali PP, Simberg D. Role of carbohydrates in the macrophage uptake of dextran-coated iron oxide nanoparticles. Adv Exp Biol Med 2012;733:115–23.

[10] Rathinam VA, Vanaja SK, Fitzgerald KA. Regulation of inflammasome signaling. Nat Immunol 2012;13:333–42.

[11] Eisenbarth SC, Colegio OR, O'Connor W, Sutterwala FS, Flavell RA. Crucial role for the Nalp3 inflammasome in the immunostimulatory properties of aluminium adjuvants. Nature 2008;453:1122–6.

[12] Demento SL, Eisenbarth SC, Foellmer HG, Platt C, Caplan MJ, Saltzman WM, et al. Inflammasome-activating nanoparticles as modular systems for optimizing vaccine efficacy. Vaccine 2009;27:3013–21.

[13] Almeida JP, Chen AL, Foster A, Drezek R. In vivo biodistribution of nanoparticles. Nanomedicine (Lond) 2011;6:815–35.

[14] Ruge CA, Kirch J, Cañadas O, Schneider M, Perez-Gil J, Schaefer UF, et al. Uptake of nanoparticles by alveolar macrophages is triggered by surfactant protein A. Nanomedicine 2011;7:690–3.

[15] Bianchi ME. DAMPs, PAMPs and alarmins: all we need to know about danger. J Leukoc Biol 2010;81:1−5.

[16] Welsh JA, Ram S. Factor H and neisserial pathogenesis. Vaccine 2008;26(S8):I40−5.

[17] Seok J, Warren HS, Cuenca AG, Mindrinos MN, Baker HV, the Inflammation and Host Response to Injury, Large Scale Collaborative Research Program, et al. Genomic responses in mouse models poorly mimic human inflammatory diseases. Proc Natl Acad Sci USA 2013;110:3507−12.

[18] Oostingh GJ, Casals E, Italiani P, Colognato R, Stritzinger R, Ponti J, et al. Problems and challenges in the development and validation of human cell-based assays to determine nanoparticle-induced immunomodulatory effects. Part Fibre Toxicol 2011;8:8.

[19] Boraschi D, Costantino L, Italiani P. Interaction of nanoparticles with immunocompetent cells: nanosafety considerations. Nanomedicine 2012;7:121−31.

[20] Donaldson K, Murphy FA, Duffin R, Poland CA. Asbestos, carbon nanotubes and the pleural mesothelium: a review of the hypothesis regarding the role of long fibre retention in the parietal pleura, inflammation and mesotelioma. Part Fibre Toxicol 2010;7:5.

[21] Liu G, Cheresh P, Kamp DW. Molecular basis of asbestos-induced lung disease. Annu Rev Pathol 2013;8:161−87.

[22] Kagan VE, Konduru NV, Feng W, Allen BL, Conroy J, Volkov Y, et al. Carbon nanotubes degraded by neutrophil myeloperoxidase induce less pulmonary inflammation. Nat Nanotechnol 2010;5:354−9.

[23] Kotchey GP, Hasan SA, Kaparlov AA, Ha SH, Kim K, Shvedova AA, et al. A natural vanishing act: the enzyme-catalyzed degradation of carbon nanomaterials. Acc Chem Res 2012;45:1770−81.

[24] Bartneck M, Keul HA, Zwadlo-Klarwasser G, Groll J. Phagocytosis independent extracellular nanoparticle clearance by human immune cells. Nano Lett 2010;10:59−63.

[25] Moghimi SM, Andersen AJ, Ahmadvand D, Wibroe PP, Andersen TL, Hunter AC. Material properties in complement activation. Adv Drug Deliv Rev 2011;63:1000−7.

[26] Moghimi SM, Wibroe PP, Helvig SY, Farhangrazi ZS, Hunter AC. Genomic perspectives in inter-individual adverse responses following nanomedicine administration: the way forward. Adv Drug Deliv Rev 2012;2012(64):1385−93.

[27] Rooijakkers SHM, van Strijp JAG. Bacterial complement evasion. Mol Immunol 2007;44:23−32.

[28] Nilsson B, Korsgren O, Lambris JD, Nilsson Ekdajl K. Can cells and biomaterials in therapeutic medicine be shielded from innate immune recognition? Trends Immunol 2010;31:32−8.

[29] Lu J, Marjon KD, Mold C, Du Clos TW, Sun PD. Pentraxins and Fc receptors. Immunol Rev 2012;250:230−8.

[30] Inforzato A, Bottazzi B, Garlanda C, Valentino S, Mantovani A. Pentraxins in humoral innate immunity. Adv Exp Biol Med 2012;946:1−20.

[31] Holmskov U, Thiel S, Jensenius JC. Collecins and ficolins: humoral lectins of the innate immune defense. Ann Rev Immunol 2003;21:547−78.

[32] Kilpatrick DC, Chalmers JD. Human L-ficolin (ficolin-2) and its clinical significance. J Biomed Biotechnol 2012;2012:138797.

[33] Vasta GR. Galectins as pattern recognition receptors: structure, function, and evolution. Adv Exp Biol Med 2012;946:21−363.

[34] Erridge C. Endogenous ligands of TLR2 and TLR4: agonists or assistants? J Leukoc Biol 2010;87:989−99.

[35] Di YP, Tkach AV, Tanamala N, Stanley S, Gao S, Shurin MR, et al. Dual acute pro-inflammatory and anti-fibrotic pulmonary effects of sPLUNC1 after exposure to carbon nanotubes. Am J Respir Mol Cell Biol 2013; (Epub ahead of print).

[36] Fadeel B. Clear and present danger? Engineered nanoparticles and the immune system. Swiss Med Wkly 2012;142:w13609.

[37] Huang YJ, Shiau AL, Chen YL, Wang CR, Tsai CY, Chang MY, et al. Multivalent structure of galectin-1-nanogold complex serves as potential therapeutics for rheumatoid arthritis by enhancing receptor clustering. Eur Cell Mater 2012;23:170–81.

[38] Lieder R, Petersen PH, Sigurjónsson OE. Endotoxins—the invisible companion in biomaterials research. Tissue Eng Part B Rev 2013;19:391–402.

[39] Lieder R, Gaware VS, Thormodsson F, Einarsson JM, Ng CH, Gislason J, et al. Endotoxins affect bioactivity of chitosan derivatives in cultures of bone marrow-derived human mesenchymal stem cells. Acta Biomater 2013;9:4771–8.

[40] ISO 29701:2010 Nanotechnologies—Endotoxin test on nanomaterial samples for in vitro systems—Limulus amebocyte lysate (LAL) test, <http://www.iso.org/iso/iso_catalogue/catalogue_tc/catalogue_detail.htm?csnumber=45640>; 2010.

[41] Li Y, Italiani P, Casals E, Tran N, Puntes VF, Boraschi D. Endotoxin contamination in nanoparticles: challenges in the use of the LAL assay. Under revision 2013.

[42] Martinon F. Mechanisms of uric acid crystal-mediated autoinflammation. Immunol Rev 2010;233:218–32.

[43] Bernstein D, Dunnigan J, Hesterberg T, Brown R, Velasco JA, Barrera R, et al. Health risk of chrysotile revisited. Crit Rev Toxicol 2013;43:154–83.

CHAPTER 3

Nanoparticles and Adaptive Immunity

Albert Duschl

Department of Molecular Biology, University of Salzburg, Salzburg, Austria

3.1 ADAPTIVE IMMUNITY—DIFFERENCES AND COOPERATION WITH INNATE IMMUNITY

Innate immunity, described in Chapter 2, is based on receptors that recognize microbial compounds (the pathogen-associated molecular patterns, PAMPs) or self-compounds that are released by necrotic cells and thus indicate acute danger (the danger-associated molecular patterns, DAMPs). The receptor repertoire for PAMPs and DAMPs is limited, with extremely little variation between individuals [1]. The receptors are present from birth and can trigger inflammatory responses without delay. Adaptive immunity, in contrast, needs several days to develop a full antipathogen response, but uses a repertoire of receptors that is highly variable and can thus recognize a virtually endless variety of stimuli. It is this flexibility that allows the adaptive immunity to attack nonself-entities that are as different as viruses, bacteria, fungi, or parasites. The adaptive immunity rests on three classes of highly variable receptors: MHC complexes, T cell receptors, and antibodies (Tables 3.1 and 3.2).

Adaptive immune mechanisms are thus in principle fully expected to recognize nanoparticles (NPs). Among the factors that determine the outcome of interaction with the immune system are NP properties like size, surface charge, hydrophobicity, and coating agents [2−4]. Engineered NPs are clearly nonself, they are often in a size range which overlaps with viruses (mostly 10−200 nm) [5], and the ability of NPs to address virus-specific pathways is indeed used in designing vaccine delivery systems [6]. Very small NPs in the size range of normal proteins (up to about 10 nm) may escape detection by the immune system, but most NPs remain monodispersed only at very low concentration. Increasing concentrations often lead to aggregation, forming structures that are well within the size range recognized by immune cells. It might therefore be expected that NPs induce immune responses as a general rule. This, however, is not the case. The reasons will be discussed in this chapter.

Due to the time delay, compared to innate immune responses, adaptive immune reactions usually occur in an environment that is already compromised and is characterized by ongoing innate immune reactions. Adaptive immunity is thus shaped—among other factors— by the type and extent of innate immune reactions present and is able to extend and enhance the already-occurring inflammatory responses. Here we may identify the first mechanism that allows us to avoid immune responses against NPs: if no innate immune receptors are triggered there are also no danger signals. Proinflammatory cytokines (TNF-α, IL-1, IL-6, etc.) are released only upon sensing danger, and nonself that fails to trigger danger receptors is tolerated [7]. Among the most important danger signals are DAMPs released from cells dying by necrosis. Any mechanism that kills cells without inducing apoptosis (including nonbiological factors) will generate DAMPs and induce inflammation. However, why should NPs kill a cell? In the absence of specific killing mechanisms, they will simply be classified as harmless by the immune system and adaptive tolerance will be established, as discussed below. Acute cytotoxicity may be induced, for example, by release of toxic ions from metal or metal oxide parti- cles. This cannot be considered to be specific immunotoxicity, but rather as general cytotoxicity, but immune parameters may be used as readouts for assessing damage.

Even if a specific NP has genuine toxic properties that can lead to cell death, these features may be attenuated after uptake into the body. Biomolecules, most prominently proteins, attach to NPs nearly immedi- ately when NPs are entering a biological matrix (e.g., sputum, lung fluid, blood, but also artificial compositions like cell culture media) forming a "protein corona" [8]. Binding of proteins may be either weak ("soft corona") or rather stable ("hard corona"). The composition of the corona depends on the proteins available in the medium and it may develop over time, even within the same medium [9–12]. Other biological molecules can bind to NPs, but proteins are usually preferred binding partners due to their variety and to the ample availability of charged or hydrophobic surface areas combined with different surface geometries.

In principle, an adaptive immune response may be directed against the NP itself, even after the attachment of biological molecules, in particular if only a "soft corona" has been formed. Alternatively, adaptive immunity may recognize nonself-proteins, if these proteins have been picked up outside of the body and derived, e.g., from microorganisms, which is not unlikely if the NPs are not clinically sterile. More worrisome are reports about responses against self-proteins (see p. 45–46), due to changes in protein structure upon binding of proteins to the NP surface. Effects on the immune system (both activation and suppression) may be due to the NPs themselves, or to larger aggregates formed by NPs, or indirectly to effects of NPs on biomolecules. In addition there may be guilt by association, when the NPs are acting as carriers for dangerous substances, like bacterial compounds or toxic chemicals carried over from synthesis [13,14].

3.2 *DE NOVO* INDUCTION OF ADAPTIVE IMMUNITY: MHC COMPLEXES AND DENDRITIC CELLS

Dendritic cells (DCs) are primarily located below all body surfaces and are often the first cells of the adaptive immune system to encounter nonself-entities entering the body. Protrusions of the DCs (dendrites) even extend to the outside of epithelia, so, for example, airways or gut can be continuously monitored. DCs take up materials from their environment and digest them. Ingested proteins are cleaved into peptides that may be degraded into amino acids, but a sizable number of nonself-peptides is loaded onto MHC complexes, and is in that form presented on the surface of the cell (Table 3.1). The human genome encompasses many different isoforms of HLA genes, which encode the MHC complex proteins. The HLA repertoire is highly diverse in all human populations, which is one of the factors explaining person-to-person variation in immune reactions [15]. If a DC takes up nonself-materials and receives additional activation signals, it leaves its site and migrates to a lymph node where it interacts with the effector cells of adaptive immunity, T and B cells.

DCs readily take up NPs, in particular if they are positively charged. For micrometer-sized polystyrene particles (1.0−4.5 μm), positively charged particles are taken up more efficiently by DCs and macrophages [16], an effect that is especially relevant for DCs that are otherwise less efficient phagocytes than macrophages. Uptake into DCs is optimal for particle sizes 500 nm and lower, while positive surface charge is aiding uptake for particles of any size [17]. It has been suggested that negatively charged NPs may be used for delivery to

Table 3.1 The Receptors/Recognition Molecules of Adaptive Immunity

NAME	FUNCTION	STRUCTURE
MHC-I	Heterodimer of a membrane spanning α-chain noncovalently linked to soluble β_2 microglobulin. Expressed on most cell types (not on red blood cells). It presents peptides coming from the cytosol (e.g., from infecting viruses) and transported to the endoplasmic reticulum.	
MHC-II	Heterodimer of membrane spanning α- and β-chains. Expressed on macrophages, DCs, T and B cells, and some epithelial cells, absent in neutrophils, red blood cells, liver, kidney, brain (except for the tissue macrophages). It presents peptides coming from endocytic vesicles (e.g., from ingested bacteria).	
TcR	The T cell receptor recognizes antigen bound to MHC and triggers T cell activation.	

Reproduced with permission from Janeway's Immunobiology, 5th Edition, Garland Science, Taylor and Francis.

DCs since positive charge leads to more unspecific uptake by other cell types [17]. However, cationic liposomes show enhanced adjuvant activity compared to anionic or neutral ones, and this is associated with the induction of T_H1 cytokines (see Section 3.3) [18]. It is not unexpected that positive NP surface charge supports uptake into cells: both phospholipids and membrane proteins are mostly negatively charged, so the surface of biomembranes should readily interact with positively charged particles. However, it should be remembered that NPs dissolved in biological liquids will quickly bind biomolecules, mostly proteins. Thus, for instance, the zeta potential of charged gold NPs in serum collapses nearly immediately toward the average value for serum proteins [8,19,20], so the cell surface should be exposed to a charge density as encountered in self-proteins—a situation that is not likely to promote specific uptake. NPs that associate proteins only transiently ("soft corona") may still have parts of their charged surface accessible to cells, but in other cases a preferred uptake into DCs would be a function of their high phagocytic potential. Alternatively, the uptake into cells may be mediated by the corona proteins, since many proteins in extracellular space (like plasma) are ligands for receptors expressed by different cells. This behavior can be used for targeting NPs to specific cell types in medical applications, as discussed elsewhere (Chapter 6).

While corona formation is interesting for delivery of drugs or vaccines, the ability of NPs to bind proteins over prolonged times raises concerns as well. Biological compounds can be acquired at different sites, including outside of the body. Among the compounds that may associate with NPs in the environment, bacterial compounds are of particular concern. Numerous bacterial compounds activate inflammatory pathways (see Chapter 2), so NPs associated with such agents will find themselves in an immune-activating context. A second class of contaminants that can be picked up by NPs outside of the body and be delivered as part of a "hard" bioshell are allergens. This type of contamination could be relevant to risk populations, that is, to allergic persons, and to persons prone to develop allergy, which may be facilitated by the codelivery of NPs and allergens. The possible effects of NPs on the development and manifestation of allergy will be covered in Chapter 4.

For safety considerations, NP effects on DCs are of concern on several levels. Cytotoxic effects of NPs may become particularly apparent in cells with high phagocytic potential. However, in a study that compared toxicity of CoO NPs and Co ions for a range of cell types, DCs were the least sensitive cell type for toxicity due to ions and the second least sensitive cell type for toxicity due to particles [21]. Both agents used in this study are clearly toxic, but it makes sense that DCs are quite resistant to toxins as such, since they are professionally taking up pathogens that can carry or release toxins (e.g., bacterial toxins like cholera toxin) but they need to be able to mature and migrate to lymph nodes or other secondary immune tissues where they activate T cells. The entire process of DC-mediated T cell activation takes several days and high sensitivity to toxins would not allow performing that function, so DCs need to be resistant to toxins.

Besides cytotoxicity, NPs may interfere with cellular functions, in particular with the intricate steps of antigen processing. How would NPs be able to disturb this process? Microbial pathogens (viruses, bacteria, fungi) contain proteins that will be processed for binding to the MHC complex. NPs do not consist of proteins, but they are associated with proteins via their bio-corona and they are able to interfere with DC activation. It has been shown that antigens delivered by biodegradable NPs can increase escape of the antigens from endosomes, resulting in efficient presentation of externally delivered antigens not only in MHC-II (as it occurs for antigens taken up from the extracellular space and going into endosomes) but also in MHC-I (as in the case of antigens free in the cytoplasm such as viral proteins) [22−24]. This process is called cross-presentation and it is important, for example, for the defense against viruses that do not infect antigen-presenting cells (APCs). Its induction by NPs shows that NPs have the potential to interfere with molecular mechanisms within DCs, thereby affecting the repertoire of peptides presented to T cells and thus modifying the adaptive immune response. The ability of DCs to recognize and present nonself-peptides and to induce specific immune responses against them has made them a major target for vaccine delivery. Many groups are working to use the specific properties of NPs to enhance uptake of vaccines and to achieve increased presentation of vaccine-derived peptides by the MHC complex (for reviews see Refs. [25,26]). Similarly, the possibility to sensitize the immune system against cancer-derived proteins using NPs both as carriers and as adjuvants has received much attention [27,28]. Some of these therapeutic options shall be discussed in Chapter 6. Immunosafety of NPs developed as drugs is reviewed in Ref. [29].

3.3 T CELL SUBTYPES

Depending on the cosignals they receive during interaction with APCs, T cells can differentiate into several different types. The cosignals involved are cell−cell contacts via adhesion molecules, and cytokines secreted by antigen-presenting and bystander cells. The context of antigen presentation thus determines the type of response, since the different T cell subsets have quite different tasks. For a simplified overview, it can be stated that T_H1, T_H17, and T_H22 cells are associated with type 1 immune response (antibacterial, antiviral, strongly linked to innate immune responses), T_H2 and T_H9 are linked to type 2 immune

Table 3.2 Activated T Cell Types	
TYPE	**FUNCTION**
Type 1 responses	
T_H1	Induction of a type 1 immune responses, critical for clearing bacteria that live within cells
T_H17	Maintenance of type 1 immune responses, leading to chronic responses, associated with autoimmunity
T_H22	Involved in chronic type 1 responses, in particular at body barriers like skin, associated with some autoimmune diseases
Type 2 responses	
T_H2	Induction of a type 2 inflammation, essential for allergic reactions, thus associated with allergy and allergic asthma
T_H9	Involved in established type 2 inflammation
Regulatory	
Treg	Immunosuppressive, down regulate both type 1 and 2 immune responses, can be already present (natural Treg) or differentiate during a response (induced Treg)
Cytotoxic	
CTL	Kill cells of the body that have been infected by viruses, also have the potential to kill other deviant self-cells, like tumor cells

response (allergic diseases and antiparasite defense), and regulatory T cells (Tregs) are responsible for suppressing immune responses and inducing tolerance (Table 3.2). For overviews of currently known and discussed T cell subtypes, see Refs. [30,31]. It has been shown in recent years that a number of cell types exist that do not express the T cell receptor or other canonical markers, but which are highly active in secreting cytokines, tentatively named innate lymphoid cells [32]. The nomenclature and identity of these novel cell types are under intense discussion, as they are in between innate and adaptive effector cells, with noncanonical T cell recognition capacity but with important regulatory capacity for adaptive immune functions (see Chapter 2). NP effects on these new cell types have not yet been studied.

A key question is whether NPs affect the expression of cytokines, since the "cytokine milieu" is essential for deciding which type of immune response will occur. Polystyrene beads coated with either the model antigen ovalbumin (Ova) or with an Ova peptide representing the minimal T cell epitope-induced T cells expressing either IFN-γ or IL-4, depending on size [33]. Size 40−49 nm was ideal for IFN-γ and size 93−123 nm for IL-4. IFN-γ is the main cytokine released by T_H1 cells, in the context of this study a preferred result, since it aimed at vaccine development where type 1 responses should be induced. IL-4 is the master regulator for type 2 reactions and is produced mainly by T_H2 cells. The different responses may be related to size-dependent preferences for uptake mechanisms, but that does not really explain the different outcomes, as both pathogen-derived antigens and allergens can be associated with particles of any size. Pulmonary exposure of mice to multiwalled carbon nanotubes (MWCNTs) induces immunosuppression linked to the production of IL-10 [34] and TGF-β [35]. Both cytokines are immunosuppressors that can be produced by several cell types, including alveolar macrophages, but they are also the signature cytokines of Tregs. A role of T cell-mediated suppression cannot be ruled out, in particular since the rise in IL-10 levels was detected in spleen [35], possibly due to Tregs that differentiated following exposure to MWCNT in the lung. These examples show that NPs can selectively affect the T_H1/T_H2 balance, thus inducing different forms of immune response, and they may also induce Treg activation, which results in immunosuppression. Immunomodulation on the T cell level is discussed in the following section.

3.4 REGULATING ADAPTIVE IMMUNITY: REGULATORY T CELLS AND ANERGY VERSUS INFLAMMATORY T CELLS

When confronted with NPs, in most cases the immune system does not react with protective mechanisms. The immune system is specialized to deal with pathogens, so its instruments are not necessarily the most suitable ones to defend the body against dangerous NPs. The induction of cell stress may be beneficial to deal with toxins and to induce apoptosis if too much damage is inflicted. In general, detoxification mechanisms promoting ejection of toxins, like increased mucus production and toxin modifications, for example, by cytochrome P450 enzymes, are professional mechanisms that protect the body from toxins. Consider that our body contains about 10 times as many bacterial cells than human cells, but nevertheless remains in healthy homeostasis. The default is to have no immune response because most nonself-agents do not harm the body. Many NPs will fall within this category. On the other hand, observing a response of the immune system toward NPs is not the same as confirming that the specific NP type is dangerous: the response may just reflect mechanisms to regain homeostasis or even active strategies to define the recognized agent as harmless.

It is not trivial to establish which T_H subset is induced by NPs. An instructive example is a study in which rats were intratracheally instilled with TiO_2 NPs that induced an initial innate immune response in the lung, followed after 1–2 days by increased levels of cytokines, including IFN-γ, IL-4, and IL-10 [36]. In other words, the signature cytokines of T_H1, T_H2, and Treg cells were all present. This is not unusual at the start of an immune response when different reactions may manifest but it clearly implies that immune events need to be followed over time to understand what is going on. In the quoted study, a type 1 response developed as late-phase response, but since the Dark Agouti rat strain used is prone to T_H1 responses, this may have been determined by the animals used. Studies in mice have reported T_H2 responses induced by TiO_2 NPs [37,38], but this could again be determined by the strains used (ICR and BALB/c mice, respectively) or it could be an effect of species difference (mice vs. rats). On the other hand, TiO_2 NPs come in different size, shape, surface area, and crystal structure, which all may also determine the type of response [39,40]. It is known that size of NPs can affect the T cell subtypes that develop, not unexpected, since size predisposes for specific routes of uptake into cells and also for more efficient uptake into different cell types, but based on available data it is not possible to draw a general conclusion which sizes would be associated with special T cell subsets [41]. Reports on selective induction of T cell subtypes by NPs should thus not be generalized without good supporting evidence, ideally based on an understanding of the molecular mechanism.

In cases where an immune response is induced, the choice of a defensive response versus tolerance is made in an interaction between DCs, T cells, and possibly other bystander cells. Importantly, tolerance is not the same as failure to recognize nonself. We recognize many nonself-entities but decide to tolerate them. The "harmless" label is maintained throughout time and rests on active mechanisms. A specific subset of T cells in charge of tolerance comprises regulatory T cells (Treg) that secrete the immunosuppressive cytokines TGF-β and IL-10. The induction of antigen-specific Tregs constitutes an active mechanism to establish and maintain tolerance, and it is one reason why we do not respond to nonself-entities like food or dust, which regularly enter our body [42]. When it is desired to ensure immune tolerance against NPs, it is a reasonable strategy to aim at obtaining active tolerance by favoring the differentiation of Tregs. Both PLGA (poly-lactic-co-glycolic acid) and

TMC-TPP (*N*-trimethyl chitosan tripolyphosphate) NPs enhance T cell activation upon nasal application. In a recent study, Ova-coated PLGA NPs applied to BALB/c mice led to differentiation of DCs that *in vitro* stimulated the differentiation of Ova-specific T cells into FoxP3$^+$ T cells [43]. NP type, charge, and size all played a role, as did the source of DCs (cervical lymph-node-derived DCs being more efficient than DCs from inguinal lymph nodes) [43]. The main message here is that the transcription factor FoxP3 is the hallmark of Treg cells. The choice of NPs can thus induce a specific type of T cells, by influencing the DCs. The differentiation of DCs depends on antigen type, dose, bystander substances, and other factors, and it leads to DC subtypes that are predisposed to induce specific types of T cells. The particles investigated here were developed for nanomedical applications [43], but it is conceivable that similar specificities exist for NPs where they are not recognized or desired. A preference for Treg induction would lead to immunosuppression, an unwelcome effect if an antipathogenic response has to be induced in cases of infection. A very direct approach to modulating the T cell subtypes induced by NPs is to load them with cytokines known to induce certain subsets. Thus, PLGA NPs loaded with the cytokine LIF induced development of Tregs, while loading with IL-6 led to increased development of T_H17 cells [44]. Importantly, the quoted study showed that neither NPs nor any of the cytokines alone reproduced the effect on T cell subtype differentiation. T_H17 cells can be seen as being nearly the opposite of Tregs [45]. While Tregs induce long-term tolerance, T_H17 cells are associated with the development of long-term type 1 reactions [46]. This type of response is important to combat pathogens that remain resident in the body for longer times, but T_H17 cells are also associated with autoimmune diseases, a detrimental form of long-lasting inflammation.

A further T cell type to be considered are cytotoxic T cells (CTL), which kill virus-infected and otherwise deviant cells, but are also producers of cytokines. Both lipid- and polymer-based NPs have been developed as adjuvants to obtain a better response to vaccination, by inducing CTL protective against viral agents [47]. A nanoemulsion based on soybean oil used to deliver thyroglobulin in a mouse model of experimental autoimmune thyroiditis led to up-regulation of Tregs and TGF-β levels and to milder disease symptoms [48]. As the human autoimmune disease Hashimoto's thyroiditis is linked to the thyroid-specific protein thyroglobulin [49], that result may lead to novel therapeutic strategies.

Besides the induction of Tregs, a second important mechanism for tolerance is permanent inactivation of effector T cells. This occurs whenever a T cell is activated with low intensity. There is no such thing as a half-activated T cell: if the activation signals are strong enough, the T cell will proliferate and become an activated effector T cell. However, if the signals received are insufficient, the activation mechanisms are shut off and the cell enters a state of anergy [50]. Importantly, anergic T cells remain in that state even if later the same antigen reoccurs combined with strong activation signals. Anergy, a state of permanent T cell inactivation, is thought to be important for tolerance against self-antigens, for example, during puberty when numerous proteins are expressed for the first time. The same mechanism could prevent defense against NPs that are usually not associated with strong immune activation signals. Both Tregs and anergy create problems when it is desired to break tolerance, for example, in the case of a tumor. A perspective for medical use of NPs is in breaking tolerance, because a tumor-specific antigen attached to an NP may possibly appear in a sufficiently different context to be recognized by new sets of T cells, thus evading both Treg-mediated suppression and tolerance due to anergy. Many types of NPs are investigated for their potential to act as adjuvants in the application of vaccines [51], and the desired induction of T_H1 responses has been shown in clinical trials [52]. The type 1 immunity induced by vaccine formulations follows an initial innate immune response, recapitulating a sequence that occurs frequently during the defense against pathogens. Inducing the same reaction in established tolerance, for example, against a tumor, would be an extremely interesting perspective.

Danger signals result when cells are damaged and release DAMPs, but other mechanisms are also possible. An extreme scenario would be that NPs themselves or the proteins attaching to them are recognized as danger signals, a case for which the term NAMPs (nanoparticle-associated molecular pattern) has been proposed [53]. This possibility is less far-fetched than it sounds, as some NPs (like carbon nanotubes) have an ordered surface, due to their synthesis procedure, in other words, a repetitive pattern, which is a type of structure that is particularly well detected by immune receptors. Ordered surfaces of NPs could also induce formation of an ordered protein layer: again a repetitive pattern.

A number of reports have demonstrated that protein binding to NPs induces conformational changes which lead to changes in biologically important properties. Selective binding of fibrinogen to poly(acryl acid)-coated gold NPs induces partial unfolding in which the D domain of fibrinogen loses its normal structure, resulting in binding to the integrin receptor Mac-1 and in induction of inflammation [54]. In this case fibrinogen turned into a DAMP; whether it also becomes immunogenic and stimulates adaptive immunity is unknown. In a further study, it was shown that the effect was dependent on the size (range 7–22 nm) of the particles used, with larger particles binding with increasing affinity and slower dissociation rate. Furthermore, in presence of excess NPs, fibrinogen induced aggregation of larger particles, consistent with interparticle bridging [55]. The proinflammatory effect of misfolded fibrinogen was most evident with small particles (5–10 nm) [54]. The complexity of the system—involving only a single protein and a single type of NP—demonstrates that it will be challenging to predict this type of interactions.

Apolipoprotein A, the major protein of high-density lipoprotein, binds to many NP types. A study investigating binding to polystyrene NPs showed effects on secondary and tertiary structure, with helical content increasing for negatively charged NPs and decreasing for positively charged ones [56]. The same study reported effects on secondary structure for reconstituted high-density lipoprotein, apolipoprotein B100, human serum albumin, and lysozyme. Absorption of carboanhydrase to silica NPs also affects the secondary structure; in that case, it is the curvature of the NP that determines the amount of perturbation to the protein' structure [57]. A study comparing five different plasma proteins (albumin, fibrinogen, γ-globulin, histone,[1] insulin) to gold NPs found conformational changes for all of them, as determined by methods including CD spectroscopy and fluorescence quenching [58]. A recent review on known examples and molecular mechanisms involved in changed properties of proteins bound to NPs summarizes the state of the art [59].

From these findings a story emerges: the body is indeed primarily exposed not to the NP surface but mostly to self-proteins. However, the proteins attached to NPs display changes in structure and possibly also in function. We are therefore dealing to some extent with an "altered self" that may induce clearance by macrophages, the normal fate of misfolded

---

[1]Histone is normally located in the nucleus of cells, associated to DNA. However, it is found at increased levels in plasma of patients with some autoimmune syndromes and neoplastic diseases.

proteins, but could also lead to new B cell epitopes (antibody-binding sites) and new T cell epitopes (peptides binding to MHC complexes): a different structure can affect how the protein is processed within the APCs. The refolding of self-proteins attached to NPs makes it an urgent matter to develop tests which can detect rather subtle modifications in the adaptive branch of immunity, like changes in the population of peptides presented in the MHC complexes of APCs. This is a challenging task due to the tremendous person-to-person variation in our adaptive immune receptors. However, the ability to change protein structure could also be turned to benefit: it has been suggested that intentional misfolding of corona proteins induced by small molecules can be applied to target NPs to specific cells for medical purposes [60]. The study showed uptake into macrophages, exploiting the recognition of the misfolded proteins on the NP surface by the scavenger receptor CD36, which is also expressed in other cell types that may be interesting for drug delivery, including adipocytes, cardiac and skeletal muscle cells, and DCs.

3.5 B CELLS AND ANTIBODIES

Soluble antibodies are secreted by activated B cells, also called plasma cells. Antibodies are expressed by naïve B cells as membrane proteins; however, upon proper stimulation they are produced in soluble form by differential splicing. Later on, excision of chromosomal DNA leads to production of different isotypes with the same recognition specificity, a process important in the development of an adaptive immune response (Table 3.3). B cell activation is usually controlled by T cells, which provide regulatory signals via cytokines and adhesion molecules, but some stimuli may result in the production of soluble antibodies in the absence of T cell help. An example is the production of antibodies against polyethylene glycol (PEG), which can be induced by PEGylated liposomes [61–64]. Repeating carbohydrates like PEG can be recognized by B cells through T cell-independent mechanisms, leading to production of soluble IgM but not of other isotypes, because class switching is strictly under T cell control. Anti-PEG antibodies are of concern, as NPs are PEGylated for therapeutic purposes, to shield the compound from the immune system. Many protein drugs are used in PEGylated form and it can be expected that NP-based drugs will have similar properties regarding possible immunogenicity of PEG. The question of PEG immunogenicity is, however, contended. Some reports claim that even in healthy blood donors, up to 25% of the

Table 3.3 Human Antibody Isotypes		
TYPE	**FUNCTION**	**STRUCTURE**
IgM	Moderate neutralization capacity, no opsonization activity, excellent complement activation. Weak extravascular diffusion. Inhibited by IL-4, IFN-γ, and TGF-β. Pentameric form.	
IgD	Membrane-bound, it acts as antigen receptor for naïve B cells. No neutralization, complement activation or opsonization activity, no extravascular diffusion. Monomeric form.	
IgG1	Good neutralization and complement activation activity, excellent opsonization capacity, and excellent extravascular diffusion. Induced by IL-4, inhibited by IFN-γ. Monomeric form.	
IgG2a	Good neutralization and complement activation activity, and excellent extravascular diffusion. Inhibited by IL-4, induced by IFN-γ. Monomeric form.	
IgG2b	Good neutralization and complement activation activity, and excellent extravascular diffusion. Induced by TGF-β. Monomeric form.	
IgG3	Good neutralization and opsonization capacity, excellent complement activation activity and extravascular diffusion. Inhibited by IL-4 and TGF-β, induced by IFN-γ. Monomeric form.	
IgG4	Good neutralization activity, moderate opsonization capacity, no complement activation activity, excellent extravascular diffusion. Monomeric form.	
IgE	Defense against multicellular parasites. No neutralization, opsonization, or complement activation capacity. It binds to parasites or allergens and triggers histamine release from basophils and mast cells. Induced by IL-4, inhibited by IFN-γ. Monomeric form.	
IgA	Defense at the mucosal level (lung, gut, urogenital tract) and in saliva, tears, breast milk. Prevention of pathogen colonization. Good neutralization activity, moderate opsonization, and complement activation capacity. Monomeric form can diffuse to extravascular sites, dimeric form can cross epithelia.	

Adapted from http://www.ufpe.br/biolmol/Aula-Imunogenetica/aula-imuno-03.htm

donors have anti-PEG antibodies [65], while a recent critical review dismissed published data on immunogenicity of PEG due to flawed and unspecific tests for anti-PEG antibodies [66].

B cells are often seen as "antibody factories." This is a useful metaphor to describe a plasma cell that produces large amounts of antibodies during infection. However, B cells are also professional APCs. Antigen presentation via the MHC-II complex instructs T cells for specific immune responses. It is not likely that NPs are able to act as T cell epitopes, that is, fitting into the peptide-binding cleft of the MHC complex.

However, NPs may interfere with the processing of antigens for MHC presentation, potentially delivering specific proteins but also affecting uptake, processing, and intracellular fate of unattached proteins. This aspect has been considered for macrophages and DCs [67,68] but has not yet been studied in depth for B cells. Of note, contact to the B cell receptor can induce a state of B cell anergy [69]. It is unknown whether NPs are able to induce such a response.

There are many studies in which NPs have been used as delivery vehicles for antigens in order to raise clinically desired antibody responses [51]. Similarly, the capacity of B cells to produce cytokines has received attention in the field [70]. Analyzing NPs as antigens is not easy since antibody binding would be most relevant in biological media (like plasma or lymph), so it is experimentally difficult to distinguish between binding of antibodies to the NP and binding to NP-associated proteins. Changes in protein structure induced by binding to NPs as discussed above, certainly do have the potential to affect the B-cell response against proteins and other biological compounds forming the NP corona in biological media. The question whether NPs can act as *bona fide* antigens remains open. Data available so far do not indicate the formation of antibodies against various NP types, maybe due to a lack of T cell help. For an overview of studies to that subject see Ref. [4]. However, even if NPs cannot act as immunogens to induce a B-cell response, they may still act as haptens (a hapten being a small molecule that can become immunogenic if linked to a larger carrier), a well-known property of fullerenes [71,72]. This may be due to the small size of fullerenes (less than 1 nm for the classical C_{60} body), but binding of anti-C_{60} antibodies to single-wall carbon nanotubes has been reported [73], so cross-reactivity is an issue. Phage display methods have been successfully used to obtain human antibody fragments binding to gold surfaces [74], but generally it is not likely that NPs without associated biological agents could induce anti-NP antibody responses in human or mice, even in presence of strong adjuvants [75].

3.6 TOXICITY AT THE LEVEL OF SPECIFIC IMMUNE CELL TYPES: DOES IT EXIST?

Immunosuppression can be achieved via toxic effects. If immune cells are depleted due to cytotoxic agents, reduced immune competence is found along with other health effects. If NPs with cytotoxic properties target specific immune cells, immunosuppression can occur even if all other cell types are present to normal levels, a situation which is most dramatically illustrated by inherited immune diseases in which one cell type is missing, for example, T cells in X-linked severe combined immunodeficiency [76]. Is it possible that toxic NPs act with similar specificity on cells of the immune system? The question is of practical interest, as genuine cell type-specific cytotoxicity would be much harder to screen with conventional cytotoxicity or viability assays, which are mostly performed in a limited repertoire of well-established stable cell lines that cannot fully represent the properties of primary cells and do not cover the complete spectrum of relevant immune cells. For primary cells, not all cell types can be obtained, and substantial person-to-person variation requires using a panel of donors, resulting in expensive and time-consuming tests.

A major selective factor for cell-specific toxicity is the preferred uptake of NPs depending on size by different types of phagocytic cells. This could, for toxic NPs, lead to a depletion of monocytes, macrophages, or DCs. T cells are specifically affected by poisons like cadmium [77], but no specific studies on T cell toxicity of cadmium-containing NPs are available. However, cadmium-containing quantum dots coupled to anti-CD4 antibodies were successfully used to label mouse T lymphocytes and spleen cells, so at least with that material there was no immediate T cell toxicity [78]. Putting the specific immunotoxicity of NPs in perspective, there are so far no reports that would firmly link NPs to the induction of either autoimmune diseases or of allergies, two types of diseases that are frequent in the population and that are associated with problems stemming from type 1 and type 2 adaptive immune reactions, respectively. NPs are investigated for treating these disorders (see Chapters 4 and 6), but no causal contribution to the development of these pathologies is known (see Chapter 5). While this question needs further investigation, NPs by themselves so far do not appear to cause specific damage to adaptive immune reactions. Preferred uptake by phagocytic cells is at this point the most likely cause for NP effects on the immune system that are not associated with overall damage to the body.

Paracelsus famously explained that the dose makes the poison,[2] but it can be added that in immunity the circumstances make the

---

[2] *Alle Ding' sind Gift, und nichts ohn' Gift; allein die Dosis macht, daß ein Ding kein Gift ist.* (All things are poison, and nothing is without poison; only the dose permits something not to be poisonous.)

poison as well. For a person undergoing an invasion of pathogens, a vigorous inflammatory response is urgently necessary, but if the same set of inflammatory agents is directed against a self-antigen, autoimmune disorders ensue. In the first case, the immunoactivating properties of certain NPs can make them useful to support therapies, for instance by acting as adjuvants to strengthen the antipathogenic response, while in the second case immunosuppressive and anti-inflammatory NPs would be in demand. If specific NPs are shown to modulate immunity in a consistent and reproducible way, this property can be considered for therapeutic application, even if the NPs were not designed for this purpose in the first place. The use of immunomodulatory NPs for medical application is addressed in Chapter 6.

REFERENCES

[1] Poznik GD, Henn BM, Yee MC, Sliwerska E, Euskirchen GM, Lin AA, et al. Sequencing Y chromosomes resolves discrepancy in time to common ancestor of males versus females. Science 2013;341:562−5.

[2] Dobrovolskaia MA, McNeil SE. Immunological properties of engineered nanomaterials. Nat Nanotechnol 2007;2:469−78.

[3] Aggarwal P, Hall JB, McLeland CB, Dobrovolskaia MA, McNeil SE. Nanoparticle interaction with plasma proteins as it relates to particle biodistribution, biocompatibility and therapeutic efficacy. Adv Drug Deliv Rev 2009;61:428−37.

[4] Zolnik BS, Gonzalez-Fernandez A, Sadrieh N, Dobrovolskaia MA. Nanoparticles and the immune system. Endocrinology 2010;151:458−65.

[5] Lipscomb MF, Masten BJ. Dendritic cells: immune regulators in health and disease. Physiol Rev 2002;82:97−130.

[6] Scheerlinck JP, Greenwood DL. Virus-sized vaccine delivery systems. Drug Discov Today 2008;13:882−7.

[7] Tang D, Kang R, Coyne CB, Zeh HJ, Lotze MT. PAMPs and DAMPs: signal 0s that spur autophagy and immunity. Immunol Rev 2012;249:158−75.

[8] Lundqvist M, Stigler J, Elia G, Lynch I, Cedervall T, Dawson KA. Nanoparticle size and surface properties determine the protein corona with possible implications for biological impacts. Proc Natl Acad Sci USA 2008;105:14265−70.

[9] Walczyk D, Bombelli FB, Monopoli MP, Lynch I, Dawson KA. What the cell "sees" in bionanoscience. J Am Chem Soc 2010;132:5761−8.

[10] Casals E, Pfaller T, Duschl A, Oostingh GJ, Puntes V. Time evolution of the nanoparticle protein corona. ACS Nano 2010;4:3623−32.

[11] Mahon E, Salvati A, Baldelli Bombelli F, Lynch I, Dawson KA. Designing the nanoparticle-biomolecule interface for "targeting and therapeutic delivery". J Control Release 2012;161:164−74.

[12] Monopoli MP, Pitek AS, Lynch I, Dawson KA. Formation and characterization of the nanoparticle-protein corona. Methods Mol Biol 2013;1025:137−55.

[13] Pfaller T, Colognato R, Nelissen I, Favilli F, Casals E, Ooms D, et al. The suitability of different cellular *in vitro* immunotoxicity and genotoxicity methods for the analysis of nanoparticle-induced events. Nanotoxicology 2010;4:52−72.

[14] Oostingh GJ, Casals E, Italiani P, Colognato R, Stritzinger R, Ponti J, et al. Problems and challenges in the development and validation of human cell-based assays to determine nanoparticle-induced immunomodulatory effects. Part Fibre Toxicol 2011;8:8.

[15] Fernandez Vina MA, Hollenbach JA, Lyke KE, Sztein MB, Maiers M, Klitz W, et al. Tracking human migrations by the analysis of the distribution of HLA alleles, lineages and haplotypes in closed and open populations. Philos Trans R Soc Lond B Biol Sci 2012;367:820−9.

[16] Thiele L, Rothen-Rutishauser B, Jilek S, Wunderli-Allenspach H, Merkle HP, Walter E. Evaluation of particle uptake in human blood monocyte-derived cells *in vitro*. Does phagocytosis activity of dendritic cells measure up with macrophages?. J Control Release 2001;76:59−71.

[17] Foged C, Brodin B, Frokjaer S, Sundblad A. Particle size and surface charge affect particle uptake by human dendritic cells in an *in vitro* model. Int J Pharm 2005;298:315−22.

[18] Peer D. Immunotoxicity derived from manipulating leukocytes with lipid-based nanoparticles. Adv Drug Deliv Rev 2012;64:1738−48.

[19] Casals E, Pfaller T, Duschl A, Oostingh GJ, Puntes VF. Hardening of the nanoparticle-protein corona in metal (Au, Ag) and oxide (Fe$_3$O$_4$, CoO, and CeO$_2$) nanoparticles. Small 2011;7:3479−86.

[20] Lundqvist M, Stigler J, Cedervall T, Berggard T, Flanagan MB, Lynch I, et al. The evolution of the protein corona around nanoparticles: a test study. ACS Nano 2011;5:7503−9.

[21] Horev-Azaria L, Kirkpatrick CJ, Korenstein R, Marche PN, Maimon O, Ponti J, et al. Predictive toxicology of cobalt nanoparticles and ions: comparative *in vitro* study of different cellular models using methods of knowledge discovery from data. Toxicol Sci 2011;122:489−501.

[22] Shen H, Ackerman AL, Cody V, Giodini A, Hinson ER, Cresswell P, et al. Enhanced and prolonged cross-presentation following endosomal escape of exogenous antigens encapsulated in biodegradable nanoparticles. Immunology 2006;117:78−88.

[23] Lee YR, Lee YH, Im SA, Yang IH, Ahn GW, Kim K, et al. Biodegradable nanoparticles containing TLR3 or TLR9 agonists together with antigen enhance MHC-restricted presentation of the antigen. Arch Pharm Res 2010;33:1859−66.

[24] Ma W, Smith T, Bogin V, Zhang Y, Ozkan C, Ozkan M, et al. Enhanced presentation of MHC class Ia, Ib and class II-restricted peptides encapsulated in biodegradable nanoparticles: a promising strategy for tumor immunotherapy. J Transl Med 2011;9:34.

[25] Kalkanidis M, Pietersz GA, Xiang SD, Mottram PL, Crimeen-Irwin B, Ardipradja K, et al. Methods for nano-particle based vaccine formulation and evaluation of their immunogenicity. Methods 2006;40:20−9.

[26] Klippstein R, Pozo D. Nanotechnology-based manipulation of dendritic cells for enhanced immunotherapy strategies. Nanomedicine 2010;6:523−9.

[27] Hung RW, Hamdy S, Haddadi A, Ghotbi Z, Lavasanifar A. Part II: targeted particles for imaging of anticancer immune responses. Curr Drug Deliv 2011;8:274−81.

[28] Hamdy S, Haddadi A, Ghotbi Z, Hung RW, Lavasanifar A. Part I: targeted particles for cancer immunotherapy. Curr Drug Deliv 2011;8:261−73.

[29] Boraschi D, Costantino L, Italiani P. Interaction of nanoparticles with immunocompetent cells: nanosafety considerations. Nanomedicine (Lond) 2012;7:121−31.

[30] Hirahara K, Poholek A, Vahedi G, Laurence A, Kanno Y, Milner JD, et al. Mechanisms underlying helper T cell plasticity: implications for immune-mediated disease. J Allergy Clin Immunol 2013;131:1276–87.

[31] Nakayamada S, Takahashi H, Kanno Y, O'Shea JJ. Helper T cell diversity and plasticity. Curr Opin Immunol 2012;24:297–302.

[32] Bernink J, Mjosberg J, Spits H. Th1- and Th2-like subsets of innate lymphoid cells. Immunol Rev 2013;252:133–8.

[33] Mottram PL, Leong D, Crimeen-Irwin B, Gloster S, Xiang SD, Meanger J, et al. Type 1 and 2 immunity following vaccination is influenced by nanoparticle size: formulation of a model vaccine for respiratory syncytial virus. Mol Pharm 2007;4:73–84.

[34] Mitchell LA, Gao J, Wal RV, Gigliotti A, Burchiel SW, McDonald JD. Pulmonary and systemic immune response to inhaled multiwalled carbon nanotubes. Toxicol Sci 2007;100:203–14.

[35] Mitchell LA, Lauer FT, Burchiel SW, McDonald JD. Mechanisms for how inhaled multiwalled carbon nanotubes suppress systemic immune function in mice. Nat Nanotechnol 2009;4:451–6.

[36] Gustafsson A, Lindstedt E, Elfsmark LS, Bucht A. Lung exposure of titanium dioxide nanoparticles induces innate immune activation and long-lasting lymphocyte response in the Dark Agouti rat. J Immunotoxicol 2011;8:111–21.

[37] Park EJ, Yoon J, Choi K, Yi J, Park K. Induction of chronic inflammation in mice treated with titanium dioxide nanoparticles by intratracheal instillation. Toxicology 2009;260:37–46.

[38] Larsen ST, Roursgaard M, Jensen KA, Nielsen GD. Nano titanium dioxide particles promote allergic sensitization and lung inflammation in mice. Basic Clin Pharmacol Toxicol 2010;106:114–7.

[39] Warheit DB, Webb TR, Reed KL, Frerichs S, Sayes CM. Pulmonary toxicity study in rats with three forms of ultrafine-TiO2 particles: differential responses related to surface properties. Toxicology 2007;230:90–104.

[40] Kobayashi N, Naya M, Endoh S, Maru J, Yamamoto K, Nakanishi J. Comparative pulmonary toxicity study of nano-TiO(2) particles of different sizes and agglomerations in rats: different short- and long-term post-instillation results. Toxicology 2009;264:110–8.

[41] Oyewumi MO, Kumar A, Cui Z. Nano-microparticles as immune adjuvants: correlating particle sizes and the resultant immune responses. Expert Rev Vaccines 2010;9:1095–107.

[42] Sakaguchi S. Regulatory T cells: history and perspective. Methods Mol Biol 2011;707:3–17.

[43] Keijzer C, Spiering R, Silva AL, van Eden W, Jiskoot W, Vervelde L, et al. PLGA nanoparticles enhance the expression of retinaldehyde dehydrogenase enzymes in dendritic cells and induce FoxP3(+) T cells in vitro. J Control Release 2013;168:35–40.

[44] Park J, Gao W, Whiston R, Strom TB, Metcalfe S, Fahmy TM. Modulation of CD4 + T lymphocyte lineage outcomes with targeted, nanoparticle-mediated cytokine delivery. Mol Pharm 2011;8:143–52.

[45] Barbi J, Pardoll D, Pan F. Metabolic control of the Treg/Th17 axis. Immunol Rev 2013;252:52–77.

[46] Muranski P, Restifo NP. Essentials of Th17 cell commitment and plasticity. Blood 2013;121:2402–14.

[47] Foged C, Hansen J, Agger EM. License to kill: formulation requirements for optimal priming of CD8(+) CTL responses with particulate vaccine delivery systems. Eur J Pharm Sci 2012;45:482–91.

[48] Wang SH, Fan Y, Makidon PE, Cao Z, Baker JR. Induction of immune tolerance in mice with a novel mucosal nanoemulsion adjuvant and self-antigen. Nanomedicine (Lond) 2012;7:867–76.

[49] Eschler DC, Hasham A, Tomer Y. Cutting edge: the etiology of autoimmune thyroid diseases. Clin Rev Allergy Immunol 2011;41:190−7.

[50] Chappert P, Schwartz RH. Induction of T cell anergy: integration of environmental cues and infectious tolerance. Curr Opin Immunol 2010;22:552−9.

[51] Smith DM, Simon JK, Baker Jr. JR. Applications of nanotechnology for immunology. Nat Rev Immunol 2013;13:592−605.

[52] Goldinger SM, Dummer R, Baumgaertner P, Mihic-Probst D, Schwarz K, Hammann-Haenni A, et al. Nano-particle vaccination combined with TLR-7 and -9 ligands triggers memory and effector CD8(+) T cell responses in melanoma patients. Eur J Immunol 2012;42:3049−61.

[53] Fadeel B. Clear and present danger? Engineered nanoparticles and the immune system. Swiss Med Wkly 2012;142:w13609.

[54] Deng ZJ, Liang M, Monteiro M, Toth I, Minchin RF. Nanoparticle-induced unfolding of fibrinogen promotes Mac-1 receptor activation and inflammation. Nat Nanotechnol 2011;6:39−44.

[55] Deng ZJ, Liang M, Toth I, Monteiro MJ, Minchin RF. Molecular interaction of poly (acrylic acid) gold nanoparticles with human fibrinogen. ACS Nano 2012;6:8962−9.

[56] Cukalevski R, Lundqvist M, Oslakovic C, Dahlback B, Linse S, Cedervall T. Structural changes in apolipoproteins bound to nanoparticles. Langmuir 2011;27:14360−9.

[57] Lundqvist M, Sethson I, Jonsson BH. Protein adsorption onto silica nanoparticles: conformational changes depend on the particles' curvature and the protein stability. Langmuir 2004;20:10639−47.

[58] Lacerda SH, Park JJ, Meuse C, Pristinski D, Becker ML, Karim A, et al. Interaction of gold nanoparticles with common human blood proteins. ACS Nano 2010;4:365−79.

[59] Shemetov AA, Nabiev I, Sukhanova A. Molecular interaction of proteins and peptides with nanoparticles. ACS Nano 2012;6:4585−602.

[60] Prapainop K, Witter DP, Wentworth Jr. P. A chemical approach for cell-specific targeting of nanomaterials: small-molecule-initiated misfolding of nanoparticle corona proteins. J Am Chem Soc 2012;134:4100−3.

[61] Judge A, McClintock K, Phelps JR, Maclachlan I. Hypersensitivity and loss of disease site targeting caused by antibody responses to PEGylated liposomes. Mol Ther 2006;13:328−37.

[62] Wang X, Ishida T, Kiwada H. Anti-PEG IgM elicited by injection of liposomes is involved in the enhanced blood clearance of a subsequent dose of PEGylated liposomes. J Control Release 2007;119:236−44.

[63] Ishida T, Wang X, Shimizu T, Nawata K, Kiwada H. PEGylated liposomes elicit an anti-PEG IgM response in a T cell-independent manner. J Control Release 2007;122:349−55.

[64] Koide H, Asai T, Hatanaka K, Akai S, Ishii T, Kenjo E, et al. T cell-independent B cell response is responsible for ABC phenomenon induced by repeated injection of PEGylated liposomes. Int J Pharm 2010;392:218−23.

[65] Garay RP, El-Gewely R, Armstrong JK, Garratty G, Richette P. Antibodies against polyethylene glycol in healthy subjects and in patients treated with PEG-conjugated agents. Expert Opin Drug Deliv 2012;9:1319−23.

[66] Schellekens H, Hennink WE, Brinks V. The immunogenicity of polyethylene glycol: facts and fiction. Pharm Res 2013;30:1729−34.

[67] Blank F, Gerber P, Rothen-Rutishauser B, Sakulkhu U, Salaklang J, De Peyer K, et al. Biomedical nanoparticles modulate specific CD4 + T cell stimulation by inhibition of antigen processing in dendritic cells. Nanotoxicology 2011;5:606−21.

[68] Shen CC, Wang CC, Liao MH, Jan TR. A single exposure to iron oxide nanoparticles attenuates antigen-specific antibody production and T cell reactivity in ovalbumin-sensitized BALB/c mice. Int J Nanomed 2011;6:1229–35.

[69] Cambier JC, Gauld SB, Merrell KT, Vilen BJ. B-cell anergy: from transgenic models to naturally occurring anergic B cells? Nat Rev Immunol 2007;7:633–43.

[70] Lund FE. Cytokine-producing B lymphocytes-key regulators of immunity. Curr Opin Immunol 2008;20:332–8.

[71] Chen BX, Wilson SR, Das M, Coughlin DJ, Erlanger BF. Antigenicity of fullerenes: antibodies specific for fullerenes and their characteristics. Proc Natl Acad Sci USA 1998;95:10809–13.

[72] Braden BC, Goldbaum FA, Chen BX, Kirschner AN, Wilson SR, Erlanger BF. X-ray crystal structure of an anti-Buckminsterfullerene antibody fab fragment: biomolecular recognition of C(60). Proc Natl Acad Sci USA 2000;97:12193–7.

[73] Erlanger BF, Chen BX, Zhu M, Brus L. Binding of an anti-fullerene IgG monoclonal antibody to single wall carbon nanotubes. Nano Lett 2001;1:465–7.

[74] Watanabe H, Nakanishi T, Umetsu M, Kumagai I. Human anti-gold antibodies: biofunctionalization of gold nanoparticles and surfaces with anti-gold antibodies. J Biol Chem 2008;283:36031–8.

[75] Dobrovolskaia MA. Nanoparticles and antigenicity. In: Yarmush ML, Shi D, editors. Handbook of immunological properties of engineered nanomaterials. Singapore: World Scientific Publishing; 2013. p. 692.

[76] Fischer A, Hacein-Bey-Abina S, Cavazzana-Calvo M. Gene therapy for primary immunodeficiencies. Hematol Oncol Clin North Am 2011;25:89–100.

[77] Lafuente A, Gonzalez-Carracedo A, Romero A, Esquifino AI. Effect of cadmium on lymphocyte subsets distribution in thymus and spleen. J Physiol Biochem 2003;59:43–8.

[78] Dong W, Ge X, Wang M, Xu S. Labeling of BSA and imaging of mouse T-lymphocyte as well as mouse spleen tissue by L-glutathione capped CdTe quantum dots. Luminescence 2010;25:55–60.

CHAPTER 4

Nanoparticles and Allergy

Albert Duschl
Department of Molecular Biology, University of Salzburg, Salzburg, Austria

4.1 ALLERGY: A SPECIAL CASE OF IMMUNE REACTION

An allergy is, according to textbook definitions, an immune-based detrimental response toward a substance that is tolerated by most people. This definition distinguishes allergens both from pathogens and toxins (detrimental to all), and it also distinguishes allergies from hypersensitivities toward physical factors like light and cold (not immune-mediated). If does not, however, restrict the definition to a specific type of immune response. The exact definition of different types of allergic reactions is complex, and, for instance, adverse responses toward drugs occur in different forms where allergies and other hypersensitivities blend into each other [1]. Rather than following these intricate discussions, we will focus here on the two types of immune response that are referred to as allergies in everyday usage: immediate-type allergies and delayed-type allergies. These two conditions are also by far the most likely to occur upon exposure to an allergenic stimulus (Figure 4.1).

Immediate-type allergies (also known as IgE-mediated allergies or type I allergies) are induced by a wide range of plant- and animal-derived proteins. They involve induction of T_H2 and T_H9 cell subsets and production of the cytokines IL-4 and IL-13. Both these cytokines induce B cells, in the presence of appropriate costimuli, to secrete IgE-type antibodies. IgE occur in blood only in minute amounts, but they are very long-lived when bound to high-affinity receptors on the surface of basophils, mast cells, and eosinophils. The long lifetime of IgE when bound to effector cells creates the problem that most allergies do not resolve, in contrast to episodes of infection that are usually over within a limited time. Re-exposure to an allergen after years or even decades can still induce allergic reactions, which puts sensitized people at risk. The incidence of allergies has increased to a shocking extent, and about 30–40% of the world population is now affected with one or more allergic conditions [2]. The majority of cases are immediate-type allergies, of which typical

	Type I	Type IV		
Immune reactant	IgE	T$_H$1 cells	T$_H$2 cells	CTL
Antigen	Soluble antigen	Soluble antigen	Soluble antigen	Cell-associated antigen
Effector mechanism	Mast cell activation	Macrophage activation	Eosinophil activation	Cytotoxicity
	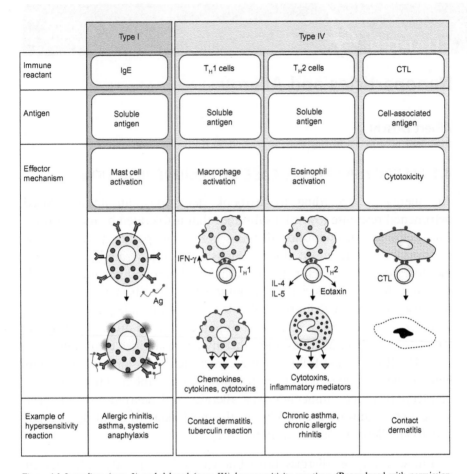			
Example of hypersensitivity reaction	Allergic rhinitis, asthma, systemic anaphylaxis	Contact dermatitis, tuberculin reaction	Chronic asthma, chronic allergic rhinitis	Contact dermatitis

Figure 4.1 Immediate (type I) and delayed (type IV) hypersensitivity reactions. (Reproduced with permission from Janeway's Immunobiology, 5th Edition, Garland Science, Taylor and Francis.)

manifestations include hay fever, house dust allergy, food allergies, and allergic asthma. If a large amount of allergens are delivered at one time, for example a bee or wasp sting, an allergic person may respond with a life-threatening anaphylactic shock, in which a systemic allergic reaction occurs. In addition, allergies of the upper airways (allergic rhinitis, better known as hay fever) can develop into allergic asthma, a life-threatening disease that can destroy the functionality of the lung.

Delayed-type allergies (also described as type IV allergies or, for most cases, contact allergies) depend on T cells, both T-helper cells and cytotoxic T cells, as well as on macrophages. As infiltration of allergen-specific cells is required, the development of an allergic response takes a few days, while immediate allergies can manifest symptoms within minutes. A well-known allergen for delayed-type allergens is Nickel, which is found in accessories like jewelry, jeans buttons, and wristwatches [3]. Allergies of this type can develop against a large variety of substances in the form of contact allergens. This is a special problem in the work place where people can be exposed to unusual chemicals over a long time, repeatedly, and at high doses. Repeated exposure over a long period of time is also the origin of contact allergies toward a range of consumer products, including toiletries and cosmetics. Concerns about contact allergies and other delayed-type allergies are focusing on work place and product safety, while for immediate-type allergies, unintentional and generally unavoidable contact with natural substances is often the case. Some allergens inducing immediate-type reactions can be avoided by sensitized persons (foods, drugs), but this is difficult for many inhaled allergens that are components of our general environment (Table 4.1). For all types of allergy, it is important to clearly separate the sensitization phase, when an allergy develops but there are usually no clinical symptoms, and the reaction phase when exposure to an allergen elicits a response.

During sensitization, IgE are produced (immediate type) or specific T cell clones are activated (delayed type). For transient exposures, the

Table 4.1 Features of Inhaled Allergens Triggering IgE Responses	
FEATURE	WHY
Carried by particles	Although soluble, allergens are often carried by particles (e.g., pollen), which probably are pivotal for favoring their interaction with the airways and lung tissues
Protein	Only proteins can trigger T cell activation, which is required in allergic reactions
Contains host-specific T cell epitopes	Allergens contain peptide sequences that can bind to the host's MHC-II molecules, thereby being able to prime specific T cell responses
Low dose	Exposure to low doses favors the activation of T cells producing IL-4 (T_H2)
Enzyme	In some cases, allergens are proteases (enabling allergens to penetrate the epithelial barrier)
Stable	Allergens are exceptionally stable (can persist unaltered in dried particles)—an important property of many food allergens that are not readily denatured in the acidic environment of the stomach
High solubility	Readily eluted from the particles
Low molecular weight	High diffusion into mucus of allergenic proteins released from the particles

allergen is often gone by the time the adaptive immune mechanisms have developed, so there are no symptoms during the sensitization phase. Without noticing anything unusual, the person has now developed an immunological memory to respond against the allergen. Thus, first exposure to an allergen usually does not induce disease symptoms. Exceptions are cases of cross-reactivity, where different antigens are similar enough to each other to be recognized as identical. For example, patients allergic to birch pollen may develop food allergy to apples, as apples contain a protein very similar to the major birch pollen allergen [4]. Note that the reverse does not occur: the apple allergen provokes reactions but does not act as sensitizing agent.

Upon re-exposure to an allergen, the anomalous immune reactions occur and cause obvious health problems. Treatment is mostly symptomatic, like the administration of histamine receptor blockers to prevent the activity of histamine, which is released by activated mast cells and basophils. The only causal therapy available is subcutaneous or oral immunotherapy, where patients receive high doses of their specific allergen in the hope to induce a shift toward a tolerant phenotype [5–7]. These therapies are often not very effective, and allergies remain a significant medical problem.

Nanoparticles (NPs) can come into play at three levels. First, they may influence the sensitization phase, making it more likely that a person responds to an allergen. Second, they may exacerbate the reaction phase, affecting the severity of the reaction. Third, they can be used as carriers or adjuvants in the development of new therapeutic principles.

4.2 NANOPARTICLES IN THE SENSITIZATION PHASE OF ALLERGY

A genuine influence of NPs on the *de novo* development of an allergy would require either an interaction with the allergen at that point or a direct effect on the immune system, promoting misdirection toward a type 2 immune response. The loading of allergen onto NPs is a mainstay of experimental therapeutic approaches (see p. 67), so the combination of NPs and allergens clearly has the potential to influence immunity, even if the NP should act only as a carrier of the allergen.

One way to explain why allergens loaded onto NPs may be treated differently from free allergens at the same dose is to consider the enrichment of allergens on the NP surface, resulting in an increased local dose. An immune cell, for example a DC, may in this way be exposed to higher allergen concentrations and, due to NPs using specific uptake mechanisms, different entry pathways into cells could be relevant as well. If allergenic proteins happen to have a high binding affinity to NPs, a "hard corona" may include them, possibly even in an ordered manner due to a patterned surface of the NP. Even NPs with a homogenous surface could induce patterning, because a shaped surface may promote binding of proteins to both this surface and to each other in an ordered way. The potential for immunogenicity increases if binding to NPs prompts changes in protein structure that expose "cryptic epitopes" [8] or if it elicits different biological effects due to altered structure (Chapter 3). If the protein in question is an allergen, this can result in a higher allergenic potential. While allergens are able to elicit responses at low ambient concentrations—one of their defining features—there are exceptions where quite high amounts of allergen are present, like seasonal plant pollen during suitable climatic conditions and animal hair in facilities that keep animals. The potential presence of "cryptic epitopes" implies of course that other epitopes may be disrupted or masked, so binding to NPs may also reduce the capacity to induce allergy (i.e., reduce the allergenicity of an allergen).

There are at present no data to demonstrate that such a specific synergy between NPs and allergens occurs, but it has to be cautioned that this may not only be due to a lack of studies aiming at that specific question, but also to the fact that it will be hard to measure it in humans, should it occur. In fact, sensitization is without clinical symptoms and it affects only a (often very small) minority of people for any individual allergen. Most people have no known allergy, despite being continuously exposed to a wide variety of allergens. It is known, however, that even small changes to proteins can strongly influence their processing in DCs and result in enhanced presentation of peptides in MHC-II complexes as well as in increased allergic responses [9].

Mouse studies in strains predisposed to develop allergies are one way to approach this problem. There are in particular numerous studies on NP effects in the Ova-BALB/c mouse model. This is a model frequently used in allergy research, because mice of the BALB/c strain will mostly respond to appropriate exposure to Ova (most commonly by intraperitoneal injection using alum as adjuvant) with a strong immediate-type allergic response [10]. There are some limitations to this model: Ova is a food allergen for humans but it is most often used in the mouse to mimic inhaled allergens, as the model can be developed to display key features of allergic asthma. The allergic response in mice differs from the human situation in various aspects. For example, while mice produce two antibody isotypes in allergy (IgE and IgG_1), humans produce only one (IgE). Most importantly, there is no phenotype in humans where all exposed persons develop an allergy—that would even exclude a reaction from being an allergy, if we consider the definition given at the beginning of this chapter. That the BALB/c mice respond so reliably in developing an allergic phenotype is very useful because it allows working with minimal numbers of animals, but it limits the correspondence to humans, in particular for the initiation phase of allergic responses.

The adjuvant alum has already been mentioned. Alum is a term that encompasses several amorphous or crystalline aluminum preparations, including hydroxide, oxyhydroxide, hydroxycarbonate, and magnesium hydroxide, all in combination with aluminum [11]. It is one of few adjuvants that are licensed for use in humans, and it supports, at least in the mouse, a T_H2-biased adaptive immune response, that is, the type that is associated with allergy. This is not a problem for human vaccine formulations that include strong bacterial or viral agents, but in mice alum is routinely used to elicit allergic responses for experimental purposes [12]. Reports on inflammatory immune responses initiated by formulations of alum and of other nanosized crystals have created considerable excitement as they have demonstrated that particles can act as danger signals, for example, by rupturing lysosomes or by direct activation of intracellular inflammation-related receptors [13–15]. These mechanisms are not limited to artificial agents, as uric acid crystals, deriving from uric acid released by necrotic cells [15,16], can also act as potent danger signals. Alum is a classic adjuvant for inducing allergic sensitization in the mouse, a property that is not fully understood but seems to be associated with its ability to induce various danger signals and to modify the expression of specific cytokines as also shown for poly(lactic-co-glycolic acid) NPs loaded with antigen [17]. Species differences have to be taken into account, as outlined above, but it is important to note that there are cases on record where NPs can specifically induce type 2 adaptive immune responses.

Delivery via air is the route of uptake for many allergens. It has been shown that some types of NPs can induce chronic inflammation in the lung, with specific parameters that are associated with allergic disease. TiO_2 NPs instilled into the lung of ICR mice induced chronic type 2 immune responses even in the absence of an allergen [18] and, together with the allergen Ova, TiO_2 NPs promoted the development of allergy in BALB/c mice [19]. Proallergic effects in mouse models have also been reported for single- and multiwalled carbon nanotubes [20−22], latex nanomaterials [23], carbon black [24−26], and for both TiO_2 and gold NPs [27].

A few caveats have to be added at this point. First, the doses used in many studies were quite high, and it is not clear that they represent any situation that can realistically occur in human exposure. Second, it is fully appreciated that significant species differences exist, and mouse data cannot be extrapolated to humans without additional controls. Third, in particular early studies were influenced by comparisons with combustion generated nanomaterials, like Diesel exhaust particles. These ambient particles are a significant problem for air quality and it is accepted that they contribute to the detrimental effects of air pollution on human health [28,29], but these unintentionally produced particles are much more complex than engineered NPs and they usually come associated with soluble and volatile chemicals, which makes it difficult to pin down the responsible mechanisms for observed effects. The nanosized fraction of environmental particles also does not seem to be acutely toxic *per se* [30].

4.3 NANOPARTICLES AND THE RESPONSE AGAINST ALLERGENS

The second phase of allergy occurs during re-exposure to allergens. Here IgE are already present (or specific T cells in the delayed-type allergies). This phase is easier to address as the patient is already sensitized, displays clinical symptoms, and will have been diagnosed by physicians to determine the relevant allergenic stimuli. What could NPs do in such a situation? This is an important question as a high percentage of the population is allergic, and it needs to be clarified whether they may require special attention as risk persons. If relevant interactions between NPs and allergens do occur, these may prompt appropriate labeling of consumer products and additional measures toward work place safety. The identification of potential risk persons is one of the present needs in nanosafety research.

In the reaction phase, NPs may act for example as an irritant in a tissue that is already inflamed. Dust will elicit a reaction when inhaled by asthmatics, and NPs, in particular if they have a propensity to aggregate, may behave similarly. An irritant effect of airborne particles could be address with antidust measures that are implemented in many working environments.

That NPs have the potential to exacerbate an already existing allergic condition is shown by animal studies. For example, nanosized SiO_2 particles lead to more severe asthmatic reactions in the lung of Ova-sensitized rats, when comparing the administration of Ova plus NPs to the administration of Ova alone [31]. In a mouse model of Ova-induced asthma, SiO_2 NPs increased allergic responses both in terms of stronger sensitization during first exposure to allergen and of stronger allergic responses during reexposure in already sensitized animals [32]. However, other studies have found that application of NPs plus allergen in already-sensitized animals reduced asthmatic symptoms, as reported for TiO_2 in Ova-sensitized rats [33,34] and for iron oxide (Fe_2O_3) NPs in mice, at least when the NPs were administered in higher doses [35].

How can some NPs reduce asthmatic symptoms? One important point is that reduced asthmatic symptoms do not equal improved health. Enhanced infiltration of neutrophils is often reported [27,34,35], and because neutrophils are typical effectors of innate immunity, this may indicate that the NPs suppress type 2 immunity by being powerful inducers of type 1 responses that are associated with innate immune system activation. When TiO_2 NPs were applied in different regimens, their effect on a mouse model of Ova-sensitization was to promote innate inflammation characterized by neutrophil immigration, when NPs were used either before sensitization or repeatedly [36]. Eosinophilia and airway hypersensitivity (hallmarks of asthma) were reduced, but other inflammation markers went up and the health of the animals deteriorated as indicated by a loss of body weight [36]: improving specific asthma parameters is not always good news.

Recent studies have aimed to clarifying molecular mechanisms by which NPs affect allergic processes in the lung. Ova-sensitized BALB/c mice showed, upon application of silver NPs, reduced levels of the growth factor VEGF (vascular endothelial growth factor) that is over-expressed in asthma and contributes to the overproduction of mucus proteins typical for the disease [37]. Signaling molecules induced by VEGF were also reduced, suggesting an effect on signaling mechanisms. In a similar mouse model, effects of silver NPs were studied at the proteomic level by collecting bronchoalveolar lavage fluid (obtained by "washing" lung sections using a bronchoscope, a technique that is also used as diagnostic procedure in humans) [38]. A number of proteins were found that were specifically present upon NP application in either healthy or allergic mice. The interpretation of the complex results obtained this way is difficult, but the advantage of "Omics" approaches is that they are hypothesis-free and allow revealing previously unsuspected connections. We can expect more studies of this type in the future.

Not all NPs enhance allergic responses. Fullerenes reduce the release of allergic mediators [39]. This sounds very positive for everybody affected by an allergy; however, the study gives rise to less sanguine interpretations. The authors have studied the IgE-dependent activation of human mast cells and basophils by a model antigen *in vitro* and found that fullerenes reduced the response, associated with an inhibition of the intracellular tyrosine kinase Syk, an enzyme that is important in immune signaling pathways. The findings could be confirmed in a mouse model [39]. For unintentional exposure, this observation is problematic because interference with signaling is one of the most challenging issues in immunology. The complex nature of signal transduction makes it extremely difficult to predict effects on the level of the organism when an inhibitor is applied, so while the report allows speculation about using fullerenes in antiallergic therapy, it is not indicating that fullerenes are harmless for immunity.

4.4 SENSITIZERS, CONTACT ALLERGY, DELAYED-TYPE ALLERGY

Delayed-type allergy is, in a sense, less serious than immediate-type allergy, as it is usually not considered to be a potentially lethal disease. However, it can lead to uncomfortable rashes and sometimes to severe skin conditions that have serious impacts on the patients (Table 4.2). Sensitization against stimuli encountered during the working activities

Table 4.2 Type IV Hypersensitivity		
PATHOLOGY	**ANTIGEN**	**PATHOLOGICAL SIGNS**
Delayed-type hypersensitivity	Proteins: insect venom, tuberculin	Local swelling (erythema, inflammatory infiltrate, dermatitis)
Contact hypersensitivity	Metal ions: nickel, chromium Haptens: dinitrofluorobenzene (DNFB), pentadecacatechol (poison ivy)	Local skin reaction (erythema, inflammatory infiltrate, vesicles, local abscesses)
Celiac disease	Gliadin	Malabsorption due to villous atrophy in small intestine

can require a change of work places, and stimuli that are also present in consumer products may force people into tiresome investigations to make sure that they are not exposed to it.

There is evidence that NPs can affect the development of skin reactions. Intravenous injection of iron oxide NPs attenuated the symptoms of delayed-type hypersensitivity in a mouse model [40], and the same was found upon application of fullerenes [41]. Interestingly, the responsible mechanisms observed in the two studies were quite different. The study on iron oxide NPs found reduced numbers of T_H1 cells and macrophages (both effectors of delayed-type allergy) but no change in immunosuppressive Tregs, while for the fullerenes, enhanced numbers of Tregs was reported, along with reduced expression of proinflammatory cytokines that are produced by the cells involved in delayed-type reactions, including T_H1 cells and macrophages.

Silica NPs aggravated atopic dermatitis-like skin lesions in a mouse model, but this effect was strongly dependent on the size of the NPs, where smaller NPs favored the development of an immediate-type response involving T_H2 cells [42]. A similar size dependency was reported for polystyrene NPs, where again smaller particles had a stronger effect in reducing symptoms of atopic dermatitis in a mouse model while up-regulating immediate-type allergy [43]. These reports make it clear that reducing skin sensitivity may not necessarily be a desired effect. If it is achieved by inducing an immediate-type allergy, the individual may be worse off. However, the induction of Tregs [41] is a promising option, as tolerance toward allergens is the general goal. The importance of sensitizers for the work place and consumer safety will keep them in focus. It is possible that in a particular work place, exposure may result in adverse responses, because the work place will often involve repeated and chronic exposure to unusual materials, potentially at high doses. The issue is closely monitored by the responsible agencies.

4.5 THERAPEUTIC PERSPECTIVES

Mostly, the best response of the immune systems to NPs is no response at all or, alternatively, the establishment of tolerance against these agents. However, if specific NPs show reproducible effects on the immune system, they may be candidates for the development of therapies. In the context of allergies, NPs are intensely investigated as carriers for allergens during specific immunotherapy, which generally aims at desensitization (induction of tolerance) by using high allergen doses. The large surface of NPs makes them ideal for carrying large loads of allergens, resulting in high local concentration of allergens, which is what is needed for therapeutic efficacy. Besides, if NPs by themselves should be are able to promote either a type 1 immune response or a tolerogenic reaction, their immunomodulatory potential is highly desired to support the redirection of immunity that is the goal for causal therapies of allergy.

Many types of NPs have been used in experimental approaches, both stable and degradable ones. The state of the art is summarized in recent reviews where specific information can be found [44–46]. Equally, the potential clinical uses as well as the problems of NPs in dermatology have been intensely investigated. For reviews see Refs. [47–49]. For the many patients suffering from allergic diseases, it is good news that NPs may offer completely new avenues for treatments, but it is remarkable that many of the materials that are now under investigation for therapeutic applications have originally been identified for having detrimental effects on immunity. As always, context is everything.

REFERENCES

[1] Barbaud A, Granel F, Waton J, Poreaux C. How to manage hypersensitivity reactions to biological agents? Eur J Dermatol 2011;21:667–74.

[2] Weinberg EG. The WAO White Book on Allergy 2011–2012. Curr Allergy Clin Im 2011;24:156–7.

[3] Hamann CR, Hamann D, Hamann C, Thyssen JP, Liden C. The cost of nickel allergy: a global investigation of coin composition and nickel and cobalt release. Contact Dermatitis 2013;68:15–22.

[4] Smole U, Wagner S, Balazs N, Radauer C, Bublin M, Allmaier G, et al. Bet v 1 and its homologous food allergen Api g 1 stimulate dendritic cells from birch pollen-allergic individuals to induce different Th-cell polarization. Allergy 2010;65:1388–96.

[5] Kim JM, Lin SY, Suarez-Cuervo C, Chelladurai Y, Ramanathan M, Segal JB, et al. Allergen-specific immunotherapy for pediatric asthma and rhinoconjunctivitis: a systematic review. Pediatrics 2013;131:1155–67.

[6] Lin SY, Erekosima N, Kim JM, Ramanathan M, Suarez-Cuervo C, Chelladurai Y, et al. Sublingual immunotherapy for the treatment of allergic rhinoconjunctivitis and asthma a systematic review. JAMA 2013;309:1278–88.

[7] Petalas K, Durham SR. Allergen immunotherapy for allergic rhinitis. Rhinology 2013;51:99–110.

[8] Lynch I, Dawson KA, Linse S. Detecting cryptic epitopes created by nanoparticles. Sci STKE 2006;2006:pe14.

[9] Karle AC, Oostingh GJ, Mutschlechner S, Ferreira F, Lackner P, Bohle B, et al. Nitration of the pollen allergen Bet v 1.0101 enhances the presentation of Bet v 1-derived peptides by HLA-DR on human dendritic cells. PLoS One 2012;7:e31483.

[10] Atherton KT, Dearman RJ, Kimber I. Protein allergenicity in mice: a potential approach for hazard identification. Ann N Y Acad Sci 2002;964:163–71.

[11] Lambrecht BN, Kool M, Willart MA, Hammad H. Mechanism of action of clinically approved adjuvants. Curr Opin Immunol 2009;21:23–9.

[12] Serre K, Mohr E, Toellner KM, Cunningham AF, Granjeaud S, Bird R, et al. Molecular differences between the divergent responses of ovalbumin-specific CD4 T cells to alum-precipitated ovalbumin compared to ovalbumin expressed by salmonella. Mol Immunol 2008;45:3558–66.

[13] Eisenbarth SC, Colegio OR, O'Connor W, Sutterwala FS, Flavell RA. Crucial role for the Nalp3 inflammasome in the immunostimulatory properties of aluminium adjuvants. Nature 2008;453:1122–6.

[14] Li H, Willingham SB, Ting JP, Re F. Cutting edge: inflammasome activation by alum and alum's adjuvant effect are mediated by NLRP3. J Immunol 2008;181:17–21.

[15] Hornung V, Bauernfeind F, Halle A, Samstad EO, Kono H, Rock KL, et al. Silica crystals and aluminum salts activate the NALP3 inflammasome through phagosomal destabilization. Nat Immunol 2008;9:847–56.

[16] Martinon F, Petrilli V, Mayor A, Tardivel A, Tschopp J. Gout-associated uric acid crystals activate the NALP3 inflammasome. Nature 2006;440:237–41.

[17] Demento SL, Eisenbarth SC, Foellmer HG, Platt C, Caplan MJ, Mark Saltzman W, et al. Inflammasome-activating nanoparticles as modular systems for optimizing vaccine efficacy. Vaccine 2009;27:3013–21.

[18] Park EJ, Yoon J, Choi K, Yi J, Park K. Induction of chronic inflammation in mice treated with titanium dioxide nanoparticles by intratracheal instillation. Toxicology 2009;260:37–46.

[19] Larsen ST, Roursgaard M, Jensen KA, Nielsen GD. Nano titanium dioxide particles promote allergic sensitization and lung inflammation in mice. Basic Clin Pharmacol Toxicol 2010;106:114–7.

[20] Nygaard UC, Hansen JS, Samuelsen M, Alberg T, Marioara CD, Lovik M. Single-walled and multi-walled carbon nanotubes promote allergic immune responses in mice. Toxicol Sci 2009;109:113–23.

[21] Inoue K, Koike E, Yanagisawa R, Hirano S, Nishikawa M, Takano H. Effects of multi-walled carbon nanotubes on a murine allergic airway inflammation model. Toxicol Appl Pharmacol 2009;237:306–16.

[22] Ryman-Rasmussen JP, Tewksbury EW, Moss OR, Cesta MF, Wong BA, Bonner JC. Inhaled multiwalled carbon nanotubes potentiate airway fibrosis in murine allergic asthma. Am J Respir Cell Mol Biol 2009;40:349–58.

[23] Inoue K, Takano H, Yanagisawa R, Koike E, Shimada A. Size effects of latex nanomaterials on lung inflammation in mice. Toxicol Appl Pharmacol 2009;234:68–76.

[24] Lovik M, Hogseth AK, Gaarder PI, Hagemann R, Eide I. Diesel exhaust particles and carbon black have adjuvant activity on the local lymph node response and systemic IgE production to ovalbumin. Toxicology 1997;121:165–78.

[25] van Zijverden M, van der Pijl A, Bol M, van Pinxteren FA, de Haar C, Penninks AH, et al. Diesel exhaust, carbon black, and silica particles display distinct Th1/Th2 modulating activity. Toxicol Appl Pharmacol 2000;168:131–9.

[26] Inoue K. Promoting effects of nanoparticles/materials on sensitive lung inflammatory diseases. Environ Health Prev Med 2011;16:139–43.

[27] Hussain S, Vanoirbeek JA, Luyts K, De Vooght V, Verbeken E, Thomassen LC, et al. Lung exposure to nanoparticles modulates an asthmatic response in a mouse model. Eur Respir J 2011;37:299–309.

[28] Heal MR, Kumar P, Harrison RM. Particles, air quality, policy and health. Chem Soc Rev 2012;41:6606–30.

[29] Anderson JO, Thundiyil JG, Stolbach A. Clearing the air: a review of the effects of particulate matter air pollution on human health. J Med Toxicol 2012;8:166–75.

[30] Hesterberg TW, Long CM, Lapin CA, Hamade AK, Valberg PA. Diesel exhaust particulate (DEP) and nanoparticle exposures: what do DEP human clinical studies tell us about potential human health hazards of nanoparticles? Inhal Toxicol 2010;22:679–94.

[31] Han B, Guo J, Abrahaley T, Qin L, Wang L, Zheng Y, et al. Adverse effect of nano-silicon dioxide on lung function of rats with or without ovalbumin immunization. PLoS One 2011;6:e17236.

[32] Brandenberger C, Rowley NL, Jackson-Humbles DN, Zhang Q, Bramble LA, Lewandowski RP, et al. Engineered silica nanoparticles act as adjuvants to enhance allergic airway disease in mice. Part Fibre Toxicol 2013;10:26.

[33] Scarino A, Noel A, Renzi PM, Cloutier Y, Vincent R, Truchon G, et al. Impact of emerging pollutants on pulmonary inflammation in asthmatic rats: ethanol vapors and agglomerated TiO$_2$ nanoparticles. Inhal Toxicol 2012;24:528–38.

[34] Rossi EM, Pylkkanen L, Koivisto AJ, Nykasenoja H, Wolff H, Savolainen K, et al. Inhalation exposure to nanosized and fine TiO$_2$ particles inhibits features of allergic asthma in a murine model. Part Fibre Toxicol 2010;7:35.

[35] Ban M, Langonne I, Huguet N, Guichard Y, Goutet M. Iron oxide particles modulate the ovalbumin-induced Th2 immune response in mice. Toxicol Lett 2013;216:31–9.

[36] Jonasson S, Gustafsson A, Koch B, Bucht A. Inhalation exposure of nano-scaled titanium dioxide (TiO$_2$) particles alters the inflammatory responses in asthmatic mice. Inhal Toxicol 2013;25:179–91.

[37] Jang S, Park JW, Cha HR, Jung SY, Lee JE, Jung SS, et al. Silver nanoparticles modify VEGF signaling pathway and mucus hypersecretion in allergic airway inflammation. Int J Nanomed 2012;7:1329–43.

[38] Su CL, Chen TT, Chang CC, Chuang KJ, Wu CK, Liu WT, et al. Comparative proteomics of inhaled silver nanoparticles in healthy and allergen provoked mice. Int J Nanomed 2013;8:2783−99.

[39] Ryan JJ, Bateman HR, Stover A, Gomez G, Norton SK, Zhao W, et al. Fullerene nanomaterials inhibit the allergic response. J Immunol 2007;179:665−72.

[40] Shen CC, Liang HJ, Wang CC, Liao MH, Jan TR. Iron oxide nanoparticles suppressed T helper 1 cell-mediated immunity in a murine model of delayed-type hypersensitivity. Int J Nanomed 2012;7:2729−37.

[41] Yamashita K, Sakai M, Takemoto N, Tsukimoto M, Uchida K, Yajima H, et al. Attenuation of delayed-type hypersensitivity by fullerene treatment. Toxicology 2009;261:19−24.

[42] Hirai T, Yoshikawa T, Nabeshi H, Yoshida T, Tochigi S, Ichihashi K, et al. Amorphous silica nanoparticles size-dependently aggravate atopic dermatitis-like skin lesions following an intradermal injection. Part Fibre Toxicol 2012;9:3.

[43] Yanagisawa R, Takano H, Inoue KI, Koike E, Sadakane K, Ichinose T. Size effects of polystyrene nanoparticles on atopic dermatitislike skin lesions in NC/NGA mice. Int J Immunopathol Pharmacol 2010;23:131−41.

[44] Broos S, Lundberg K, Akagi T, Kadowaki K, Akashi M, Greiff L, et al. Immunomodulatory nanoparticles as adjuvants and allergen-delivery system to human dendritic cells: implications for specific immunotherapy. Vaccine 2010;28:5075−85.

[45] De Souza Reboucas J, Esparza I, Ferrer M, Sanz ML, Irache JM, Gamazo C. Nanoparticulate adjuvants and delivery systems for allergen immunotherapy. J Biomed Biotechnol 2012;2012:474605.

[46] Craparo EF, Bondi ML. Application of polymeric nanoparticles in immunotherapy. Curr Opin Allergy Clin Immunol 2012;12:658−64.

[47] Wiesenthal A, Hunter L, Wang S, Wickliffe J, Wilkerson M. Nanoparticles: small and mighty. Int J Dermatol 2011;50:247−54.

[48] Choksi AN, Poonawalla T, Wilkerson MG. Nanoparticles: a closer look at their dermal effects. J Drugs Dermatol 2010;9:475−81.

[49] Papakostas D, Rancan F, Sterry W, Blume-Peytavi U, Vogt A. Nanoparticles in dermatology. Arch Dermatol Res 2011;303:533−50.

CHAPTER 5

Nanoparticles and Immunological Frailty

Diana Boraschi
CNR, Institute of Protein Biochemistry, Napoli, Italy

5.1 WHEN DOES IMMUNOLOGICAL FRAILTY OCCUR?

Immunological frailty encompasses all the diverse situations in which the immune response is not adequate (Table 5.1). An example that is universally known is that of AIDS patients who, because of the selective killing of T cells by the virus, become susceptible to many different kinds of infections and often die due to infections by microorganisms that are normally considered as harmless. In fact, these patients become infected with microorganisms that rarely succeed in causing an infection in normal people, due to the fact that the patient's immune system is unable to protect them against such agents. This underlines the notion that our well-being is the result of a constantly active immune surveillance.

When and how can the immune system fail? There are several possibilities. **Newborn babies**, for instance, have an immature immune system. It takes about 1 year for full development, a reason why babies are more susceptible to a series of diseases. Infections such as measles can kill babies below 1 year of age, while it rarely kills those above that age. Immunity to polysaccharides does not develop until a few years of age, which poses a problem for several polysaccharide-based vaccines that are not effective in young children. For some devastating infections of the newborn (such as the deadly Group B *Streptococcus*), vaccinating the mothers is by now seen as the best way for protecting the child.

Pregnant women also have altered immunity. The reason is that the developing fetus may be considered a sort of allotransplant (similar to a noncompatible organ), and therefore the immune system of the mother needs to avoid a "rejection" response, triggered by the fetal nonself proteins provided by the father's DNA. On the other hand,

Table 5.1 Immunological Frailty: Population Groups at Risk		
GROUP	CAUSE OF IMMUNOLOGICAL FRAILTY	EXPECTED CONSEQUENCE ON HEALTH
Age		
Newborns and infants (below 1 year)	Immunological immaturity	Susceptibility to infections, often with severe consequences
Young children (below 5 years)	Immunological immaturity	Lack of responsiveness to certain agents (e.g., polysaccharides), with consequent inadequate reaction to some infections
Elderly (> 65 years)	Immunological senescence	Slower and lower reaction to certain agents, with increased susceptibility in particular to respiratory diseases
Life Conditions		
Malnutrition (insufficient)	General and immunological weakening	Increased susceptibility to all kinds of dangerous events (infections, tumors, etc.), slower capacity of recovery
Malnutrition (obesity)	Low grade chronic inflammation	Anomalous reactivity to danger, increased incidence of infections and other diseases (metabolic syndrome, tumors, cardiovascular and respiratory illnesses, diabetes)
Stress (in particular when chronic)	Generalized immunosuppression	Increased susceptibility to all kinds of dangerous events (infections, tumors, etc.)
Diseases and Drugs		
Immunosuppressive drugs	Generalized immunosuppression	Increased susceptibility to all kinds of dangerous events (infections, tumors, etc.)
Infections (e.g., AIDS)	Generalized immunosuppression	Increased susceptibility to all kinds of dangerous events (infections, tumors, etc.)
Tumors	Generalized immunosuppression	Increased susceptibility to all kinds of dangerous events (infections, tumors, etc.)
Allergy and asthma	Immune hyperreactivity	Exaggerated reaction to usually harmless agents
Autoimmunity	Immune hyperreactivity	Reaction to self-molecules, chronic tissue, and organ damage

because it is very important that the mother stays in good health in order to carry out successfully her pregnancy, the immune system is highly active in keeping off dangerous agents. Immunity during pregnancy is a particularly complex issue, but in any case, despite the lack of rejection of the fetus, it is obvious that there is no generalized immunosuppression, and therefore no classical frailty [1].

Malnutrition is an extremely important cause of immunological frailty. While this is an infrequent problem in developed countries, malnourished people are very frequent in Sub-Saharan Africa and in other less-developed areas. The reasons for inadequate immunity in malnourished people are obvious, being linked to the general weakening of the entire organism: the correlation between body mass index (BMI: kg/m^2) and death for infections is striking, with risk increasing five times with a BMI below 15 [2]. Malnutrition in developed countries is usually associated with old age, as we will see (Section 5.3). On the other hand, immunological inadequacy also accompanies obesity, in which a constant inflammatory status increases the susceptibility to infections [3].

Another long-known cause of immunosuppression is **stress**, in particular when it becomes a chronic disease state. Indeed, **disease** is among the most frequent and widespread causes of immunological frailty together with **aging**. Both will be described below (Sections 5.2 and 5.3).

5.2 DISEASE

We can group diseases in those that cause immunosuppression and those that imply immunological hyperreactivity.

Diseases that cause immunosuppression, directly or indirectly, are infections and tumors. In the case of the HIV-1 infection that causes AIDS, the selective killing of $CD4^+$ T lymphocytes by the virus causes a generalized immunosuppression, whereby the organism becomes unable to properly react to a large variety of microbes or unable to counteract the development of tumors. Indeed, it is noteworthy that AIDS patients can be infected and also killed by microorganisms that are harmless to healthy people or develop tumors such as the Kaposi sarcoma that rarely occur in immunologically competent people [4].

Besides the extreme and well-known case of HIV-1, strategies for escaping or suppressing immune responses have been developed by all successful infectious microorganisms, as circumventing immunity is their winning survival strategy (see for instance Ref. [5]). It is interesting to note, in this respect, that our coexistence with bacteria (the "microbiota"; in the human body there are 10 bacteria for each human cell) is actively regulated by our immune system at the interfaces between host and external environment. In the gut, where the majority of our bacteria are located, mucosal production of the cytokine IL-18 is apparently key to keeping bacteria in check, with commensal bacteria becoming invasive if IL-18 is missing [6].

Tumors, similarly to microorganisms, can develop only if they are able to circumvent the immune surveillance and antitumor immune effectors. Thus, tumors can produce anti-inflammatory and immunosuppressive molecules or, in the case of solid tumors, re-educate incoming inflammatory leukocytes (such as macrophages) from tumoricidal cells to anti-inflammatory cells with angiogenic and tissue reconstruction capacity, thereby exploiting them for their own growth and expansion [7].

Diseases such as allergies (see Chapter 4), degenerative, chronic inflammatory, and autoimmune diseases (multiple sclerosis, rheumatoid arthritis, inflammatory bowel diseases, systemic lupus erythematosus, etc.) are all based on anomalous immune reactivity (reactivity to usually harmless agents or to self-antigens) or exaggerated immune reactivity (excessive, persistent/chronic responses). Many of these diseases imply abnormal inflammation, with activated leukocyte and inflammatory cytokines becoming the cause of the physical and functional tissue damage. Therapy with inflammatory cytokine inhibitors, as in the case of anti-TNF-α and anti-IL-1β drugs (antibodies or antagonists), leads to significant symptom alleviation in many of these diseases, underlining the central pathological role of abnormal innate immunity/inflammation in these syndromes [8,9].

It should be mentioned here that in people with tumors, infections, autoimmune diseases, or organ transplants, an additional cause of immunological frailty is the therapy with anti-inflammatory and immunosuppressive drugs: corticosteroids, cyclosporine, chemotherapeutics, biologics such as anti-TNF-α all have immunosuppressive effects and can promote the susceptibility of the patient to opportunistic infections and other kinds of aggression.

5.3 AGING

Prolongation of life expectancy is causing the rapid aging of the world population, both in developed and developing countries. By the year 2030, the population that will have ≥ 60 years of age is predicted to represent over 25% of the total population, of which 75% will be living in less-developed countries. Thus, a major public health challenge in the twenty-first century is how to ensure healthy and active aging ("adding life to years" is the motto of WHO for healthy aging actions).

The aging of the immune system is the objective of active research, in order to devise strategies for immune "rejuvenation" that will ensure better reaction to infections, which are indeed the major cause of morbidity and mortality in the elderly and in developed countries [10]. The elderly immune system is generally characterized by a reduced frequency of naïve immune cells and by increased, and therefore already biased, memory cells. This is why elderly people may be better protected as opposed to younger people against some pandemic infections (which they have already encountered in their life). On the other hand, the relative inability to recognize novel infections and the generally less adequate capacity of reacting makes them more susceptible to diseases, in particular to respiratory illnesses. Moderate physical exercise, constant intellectual stimulation, good nutrition, and prevention (vaccination) are among the actions that can delay immune aging and the transition from "young old" to "old old" [10]. In fact, immunological frailty in the elderly is not only due to age, but it is the summing-up of several risk factors, including disease and malnutrition. An example is that of periodontal diseases, very frequent in the elderly, which can cause malnutrition due to tooth loss and consequent difficulties in feeding, and that contribute to both respiratory and cardiovascular problems and to chronic inflammatory diseases such as diabetes and rheumatoid arthritis [11,12].

5.4 INTERACTION OF NANOPARTICLES WITH FRAIL IMMUNE SYSTEMS

Immunological frailty is a particularly important risk factor when examining the possible effects of NPs on human health. For example, as for other kinds of insults, inhalation of high dosages of SiO_2 NPs caused more severe cardiopulmonary disorders in old rats as compared to young animals [13], while high dosages of metal NPs showed more pronounced neurotoxicity in very young or very old rats as compared to adult animals [14]. Although the role of frail immunity has not been fully investigated in these circumstances, it is conceivable that to the local damage could concur the anomalous capacity of the immune system to deal with the foreign particles. While in the case of old age, cardiopulmonary diseases or cancer, the issue is an impaired capacity to eliminate the particles, in other diseases the presence of NPs may cause enhanced reaction.

The majority of information available of how NPs can exacerbate an underlying disease status relates to respiratory syndromes, in particular allergies and allergic asthma (see Chapter 4). Indeed, it is intuitive to expect that inhalations of NPs into an already inflamed lung tissue may lead to increased distress and exacerbate the disease. In the case of autoimmune diseases, a role of NPs in disease initiation has been long hypothesized, however there is no formal proof of it. Recently, SiO_2 NPs and carbon nanotubes were shown to increase protein citrullination *in vitro* and *in vivo*, suggesting a possible contribution to the pathogenesis of rheumatoid arthritis, in which autoantibodies to citrullinated self proteins are a hallmark [15]. In any case, given the particularly complex multifactorial origin of autoimmune diseases, which includes genetic and nongenetic elements and a strong involvement of the microbiota, if NPs contribute to disease development or exacerbation they may do it not only by providing an additional challenge to the immune system that contributes to amplifying the chain of anomalous pathological events, but also by interfering with the microbiota homoestasis leading to immune dysfunction [16]. The concept that health depends on the cross talk between our immune system and our commensal microbiota, will open important new directions in understanding the safety of nanomaterials.

Thus, whereas little is known about the susceptibility of immunologically frail people to the putative detrimental effects of NPs, it is likely that these population groups are more at risk than immunocompetent adult healthy people, in line with the known increased susceptibility to infections and tumors. This would suggest that the nanosafety studies should be targeted in particular to immunocompromised and immunologically altered people, as effects may be identified that do not occur in the "normal" population.

REFERENCES

[1] Mor G, Cardenas I. The immune system in pregnancy: a unique complexity. Am J Reprod Immunol 2010;63:425–33.

[2] Flicker L, McCaul KA, Hankey GJ, Jamrozik K, Brown WJ, Byles JE, et al. Body mass index and survival in men and women aged 70 to 75. J Am Geriatr Soc 2010;58:234–41.

[3] Milner JJ, Beck MA. The impact of obesity on the immune response to infection. Proc Nutr Soc 2012;71:298–306.

[4] Harden VA. AIDS at 30: a history. Dulles, VA: Potomac Books Inc.; 2012.

[5] Alcami A, Koszinowski UH. Viral mechanisms of immune evasion. Immunol Today 2000;21:447−55.

[6] Elinav E, Strowig T, Kau AL, Heneo-Mejia J, Thaiss CA, Booth CJ, et al. NLRP6 inflammasome regulates colonic microbial ecology and risk for colitis. Cell 2011;145:745−57.

[7] Mantovani A, Sozzani S, Locati M, Allavena P, Sica A. Macrophage polarization: tumor-associated macrophages as paradigm for polarized M2 mononulcear phagocytes. Trends Immunol 2002;23:549−55.

[8] Feldmann M, Williams RO, Peleolog E. What have we learnt from targeted anti-TNF therapy?. Ann Rheum Dis 2010;69:i97−9.

[9] Dinarello CA, Simon A, van der Meer JWM. Treating inflammation by blocking interleukin-1 in a broad spectrum of diseases. Nat Rev Drug Discov 2012;11:633−52.

[10] Boraschi D, Aguado MT, Dutel C, Goronzy J, Louis J, Grubeck-Loebenstein B, et al. The gracefully aging immune system. Sci Transl Med 2013;5:185ps8.

[11] Bansal M, Rastogi S, Vineeth N. Influence of periodontal disease on systemic disease: inversion of a paradigm: a review. J Med Life 2013;6:126−30.

[12] Detert J, Pischon N, Burmester GR, Buttgereit F. The association between rheumatoid arthritis and periodontal disease. Arthritis Res Ther 2010;12:218.

[13] Chen Z, Meng H, Xing G, Yuan H, Zhao F, Liu R, et al. Age-related differences in pulmonary and cardiovascular responses to SiO_2 nanoparticle inhalation: nanotoxicity has susceptible population. Environ Sci Technol 2008;42:8985−92.

[14] Sharma A, Muresanu DF, Patnail R, Sharma HS. Size- and age-dependent neurotoxicity of engineered metal nanoparticles in rats. Mol Neurobiol 2013;2013;48:368−79.

[15] Mohamed BM, Verma NK, Davies AM, McGowan A, Crosbie-Staunton K, Prina-Mello A, et al. Citrullination of proteins: a common post-translational modification pathway induced by different nanoparticles *in vitro* and *in vivo*. Nanomedicine (Lond) 2012;7:1181−95.

[16] Fung I, Garrett JP, Shahane A, Kwan M. Do bugs control our fate? The influence of the microbiome on autoimmunity. Curr Allergy Asthma Rep 2012;12:511−9.

CHAPTER 6

Nanoparticles in Medicine: Nanoparticle Engineering for Macrophage Targeting and Nanoparticles that Avoid Macrophage Recognition

S. Moein Moghimi[1] and Z. Shadi Farhangrazi[2]

[1]Nanomedicine Research Group, Centre for Pharmaceutical Nanotechnology and Nanotoxicology, University of Copenhagen; Denmark and NanoScience Centre, University of Copenhagen, Copenhagen, Denmark [2]Biotrends International, Denver Technology Center, Greenwood Village, CO

6.1 INTRODUCTION

Particulate systems of various sizes and shapes (e.g., liposomes, oil-in-water emulsions, polymeric nano- and microspheres, metallic nanoparticles (NPs) such as gold, silver, and iron oxide crystals, core-shell hybrid NPs) offer many diagnostic and therapeutic applications (Figure 6.1; Table 6.1) [1,2]. For instance, small and large molecule therapeutics can be encapsulated in liposomes and polymeric particles. One advantage of encapsulation strategy is to afford protection against drug degradation or inactivation en route to the target site. Furthermore, drug encapsulation may reduce the amount of active agent needed to obtain a beneficial therapeutic effect and effectively minimize or eliminate drug-induced toxicity. Drug encapsulation in particulate carriers may be considered a viable approach for selection and administration of highly potent drugs that have previously been discarded on the grounds of high toxicity, poor solubility, and instability in the systemic circulation [2]. However, therapeutic molecules entrapped in a particulate carrier are not bioavailable unless released. Accordingly, the pharmacokinetic parameters of the encapsulated drugs will be controlled by physicochemical properties of the carrier that regulate drug release and biological factors that modulate carrier performance (e.g., stability, circulation times, biodistribution) [1,2]. Particulate carriers, however, by virtue of their size, shape, and surface properties (e.g., display of structures with repeated domains) may resemble many microorganisms. These properties make particulate carriers prone for interception by different components of the body's defenses following entry into the body [3,4]. Accordingly, the type and

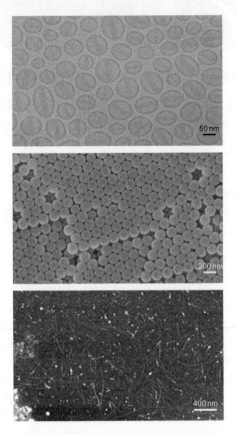

Figure 6.1 Examples of NPs in medicine. Cryo-transmission electron micrographs of single unilamellar vesicles with entrapped doxorubicin (top image), scanning electron micrographs of polymeric nanospheres (middle image), and atomic force microscopy images of single-walled carbon nanotubes coated with poly(ethylene glycol)$_{5000}$--phospholipid conjugates (bottom image).

the extent of immune responses will depend on physicochemical characteristics of the carrier, administered dose, frequency of administration, and the portal of entry.

Immune responses frequently comprise safe elimination and destruction by phagocytic cells, as discussed in Chapter 2 [3–5]. This, however, offers an unprecedented opportunity for delivery of therapeutic agents to these cells (Table 6.2) [6]. Examples include delivery of antimicrobials (because macrophages serve as the site of proliferation for many pathogens), metabolic enzymes for enzyme-replacement therapy (e.g., glucocerebrosidase), and even toxins (for selective macrophage elimination in relation to specific pathological conditions) [6]. The macrophage

Table 6.1 Selected Examples of NPs in Medicine

NP COMPOSITION	EXAMPLES	APPLICATIONS
Lipid-based	Liposomes: vesicular structures consisting of amphiphilic lipid forming bilayer enclosing part of the aqueous phase in which they are dispersed. Liposomes have different morphologies and sizes. Examples include multilamellar vesicles, small unilamellar vesicles, large unilamellar vesicles, and giant unilamellar vesicles.	Delivery of therapeutic (e.g., drugs, enzymes, antigens, nucleic acids) and diagnostic agents.
Polymer-based	Nanospheres: this refers to polymer-based structures where the pharmaceutical agents are dispersed throughout the structure. Nanocapsules: these structures are composed of an oily or an aqueous drug-containing core surrounded by a polymeric membrane.	Similar to liposomes.
Inorganic NPs	Gold, Quantum dots, iron oxide.	Medical imaging (computed tomography, fluorescent, magnetic resonance).
Carbon NPs	Single-walled carbon nanotubes, multiwalled carbon nanotubes; fullerene.	Delivery vehicles, Contrast agents (magnetic resonance, ultrasound).
Composite NPs	Core-shell NPs (silica-gold); carbon nanotube–iron oxide hybrids.	Photothermal abalation of pathological cells (e.g., tumor cells) under magnetic resonance guidance.

Table 6.2 Applications of NPs in Macrophage Targeting

PATHOPHYSIOLOGICAL CONDITION	EXAMPLE
Infectious diseases (macrophage infections)	Bacterial: Tuberculosis (antibiotic and immunomodulator delivery)
	Fungal: Leishmaniasis (delivery of antimonial drugs and immunomodulators)
	Viral: Rift valley fever virus (delivery of immunomodulators/ lymphokines)
Macrophage storage/metabolic diseases	Gaucher's disease (enzyme-replacement therapy: delivery of glucocerebroside β-glucosidase)
Macrophage neoplastic diseases	Histiocytosis X (delivery of cytotoxic agents)
Autoimmune and inflammatory conditions with macrophage involvement	Autoimmune blood disorders, spinal cord injury, restonosis, rheumatoid arthritis (macrophage "suicide" approaches)
Disease diagnosis through macrophage involvement	Macrophage loading with contrast agents (e.g., for detection of atherosclerosis, rheumatoid arthritis, lymph node mapping)
Host protection through macrophage involvement	Vaccination (antigen delivery to macrophages and antigen-presenting cells)

phagocytic/endocytic pathway will direct nanoparticulate drug carriers to lysosomes, where local degradation processes will release the entrapped cargo from the carrier into phagosome-lysosome vesicles. Efficient cargo delivery to cytosol, however, may be achieved by triggered release mechanisms in late endosomes. Examples include pH-sensitive and fusogenic drug carriers [7].

Moreover, particulate systems may be used as immune potentiators or adjuvants triggering elements of innate immunity that subsequently assist the generation of potent and persistent adaptive immune responses [8]. Indeed, a wide range of organic and inorganic particulate systems are receiving attention as adjuvants for vaccine formulations [8–10]. Most of these efforts are being directed to enhance the immunogenicity of subunit vaccines through both antigen protection and targeting to antigen-presenting cells as well as immunostimulation [8–10]. The latter may involve complement system (for instance some complement activation products can induce B-cell activation) or direct activation of NALP3 inflammasome complex (apoptosis-associated speck-like protein and caspase-1 protease), which in turn cleaves and activates the immunostimulatory cytokine IL-1β [10,11].

Rapid interception and elimination of particulate carriers by phagocytic cells, however, is of concern if the intended target site for therapeutic intervention lies elsewhere [2]. However, many pathogens have deployed strategies that overcome interception by body's defenses at many levels [5]. Understanding of these strategies has provided means for design and engineering of "phagocyte-resistant" particulate drug carriers and functional nanosystems [5]. Fundamentals of macrophage interception of particulate matters and in relation to therapeutic particle design are discussed in this chapter.

6.2 MACROPHAGE DISTRIBUTION, ACTIVATION, AND HETEROGENEITY

Macrophages are widely distributed and strategically placed in many tissues and in different body compartments, which allow them to readily intercept particulate invaders (Figure 6.2) [12]. In the vascular compartment, the hepatic macrophages (Kupffer cells) are the predominant scavengers and constitute the largest population of macrophages in direct contact with the blood in human, mice, and rats

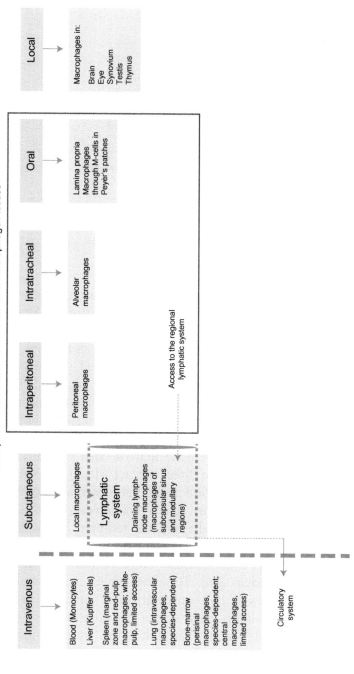

Figure 6.2 *NPs can reach macrophages through different portals of entry.*

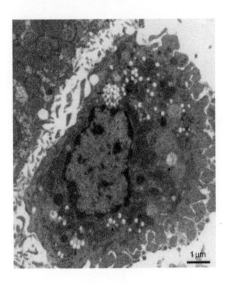

Figure 6.3 An electron micrograph of a rat Kupffer cells with ingested polymeric NPs localized in lysosomal compartments.

(Figure 6.3) [6]. Hepatic macrophages have been classified according to their location and phenotype. Among them, the periportal Kupffer cells, comprising 45% of total liver macrophages, exhibit high scavenging abilities, which is also reflected in their larger size and higher lysosomal enzyme activity (on a per cell basis), compared with Kupffer cells located in the hepatic midzonal and perivenous regions [13]. In species such as calves, pigs, cats, goats, and sheep, the main scavenging role is assigned to pulmonary intravascular macrophages that are adherent junctionally to the capillary endothelium of lungs [14]. Organs such as the spleen and the bone marrow also contain some macrophage populations that are in direct contact with the blood and can participate in particle extraction from the systemic circulation [15,16]. In the human and the rat spleen (examples of sinusoidal spleens), these include marginal zone and the red-pulp macrophages [15]. In some species such as rabbits (but not humans), macrophages also appear in the sinuses of bone marrow—blood barrier and these are termed perisinal macrophages [16]. However, access to stromal or hematopoietic macrophages of the bone marrow is typically through transcellular and intercellular passage across the bone marrow sinus endothelium [16]. Monocytes (and other leukocytes) are scavengers in the blood, but due to their low numbers relative to Kupffer cells, their scavenging role is marginal [6]. Some particles, depending on their physiochemical properties, may reach macrophages located at pathological sites such as solid tumors and atherosclerotic plaques [1,2,5].

On intraperitoneal route of entry, peritoneal phagocytes will intercept a large fraction of particles, but some particles could reach macrophages in the lymph nodes through stomata in the diaphragm [17]. Local interstitial macrophages as well as dendritic cells (DCs) (interstitial and dermal DCs, Langerhans cells) will confront particles present at subcutaneous sites [10,18]. A significant fraction of the particles at interstitial spaces, again depending on their physicochemical properties, may drain into the initial lymphatic system and be conveyed to the regional draining lymph nodes for extraction by macrophages located at the subcapsular floor and medullary sinuses [18−20]. Lymph node sinus-resident immature DCs may also participate in particle clearance [18]. Alveolar macrophages are strategically placed to intercept air-borne particles [6]. In contrast to these, only a small fraction of particulate matters may ever reach phagocytes located in the brain, gut, testis, synovial cavity, and the eye, unless administered locally into these sites. In the gut, some particles may gain access to macrophages and DCs of the *lamina propria* through the M cells of the Peyer's patches [21]. Macrophages are very flexible cells that react to surrounding stimuli by initiating one of several activation programs. Historically, they have been classified into two main groups designated M1 and M2 [22]. M1 macrophages are immune effector cells that engulf and digest pathogens and various particles. M1 macrophages are activated by bacterial lipopolysaccharides and interferon-γ. They secrete high levels of IL-12 but low levels of IL-10. M1 activity inhibits cell proliferation and causes tissue damage [22]. M2 macrophages are alternatively activated macrophages. Generally, they are activated by IL-4, produce high levels of IL-10 and low levels of IL-12. M2 macrophages promote cell proliferation and tissue repair [22]. Tumor-associated macrophages are thought to be M2 macrophages [22]. Macrophages display remarkable heterogeneity even within the same tissue [23−27]. For example, functional and phenotypic heterogeneity are evident in the mouse spleen where there are at least five different subpopulations of macrophages [26]. Functional and phenotypic heterogeneity has also been noted in both rat and human Kupffer cell populations [27]. Circulating monocytes, which give rise to mature macrophages, are also heterogeneous [25]. The different monocyte subsets may reflect developmental stages with distinct physiological roles.

6.3 MACROPHAGE RECOGNITION OF NANOPARTICLES

Macrophages express an extensive receptor repertoire that equips them for rapid recognition and clearance of a wide range of particulate matters [6,12]. These include the family of scavenger receptors, Toll-like receptors, carbohydrate receptors (mannose receptor, fucose/galactose receptor), complement receptors, Fc receptors, tuftsin receptor, and Dectins. These receptors recognize various features on particles either directly or through opsonization processes in plasma, lymph, and tears [1,2,5,6]. Accordingly, particulate targeting of macrophages may be improved through surface modification with macrophage receptor ligands such as mannose and tuftsin [1,6]. Key opsonic molecules include complement proteins such as C1q, C3-derived species (e.g., C3b and iC3b), antibodies (notably IgG and IgM isotypes), and fibronectin [1,2]. Particles of different physicochemical properties may attract different arrays of opsonins. These processes may not only control which subpopulation of macrophages will host the particles but could also indicate a recognition hierarchy phenomenon in phagocytic clearance [6]. Nevertheless, the complement system and complement proteins play a key role in particle recognition and clearance by macrophages [2,28]. For example, both negatively- and positively-charged liposomes activate and fix complement proteins considerably more than zwitterionic vesicles [29]. The pathways of complement activation have also been shown to be different between liposomes of different lipid composition and electric charges [29]. Some anionic vesicles activate the classical pathway of complement purely by binding C1q, which is attributed to the pattern recognition property of C1q arising from its cationic globular head. Liposome-mediated complement activation may further be dependent on the binding of naturally-occurring antibodies to phospholipid head groups and cholesterol [29]. For example, each globular head of C1q can bind to the Fc region of immunoglobulin; the CH2 domain of IgG, or the CH3 domain of IgM, but multivalent attachment of C1q is required for C1 activation. As IgG is monomeric, at least two molecules are required to cross-link the globular head of C1q and activate C1. On a typical surface, two IgG molecules must be within 10– 40 nm of each other to form a stable binding site for C1q. On the other hand, a single pentameric IgM is sufficient to activate C1, which allows at least two C1q heads to bind to separate Fc pieces. Human IgM is a mushroom-shaped complex with a central 20 nm circular region and 11 nm radial arms.

When deposited on NPs of similar dimensions (e.g., 40– 60 nm), IgM becomes geometrically strained and this conformational change is sufficiently enough to allow C1q accommodation and activation of the classical pathway of the complement [30].

Particle shape can also modulate the specificity of antibody-displaying NPs. For example, antibody-coated rod-shaped particles exhibit higher specific uptake and lower non-specific uptake in cells compared with spherical counterparts [31]. Accordingly, shape-induced enhancement of antibody specificity and avidity (accumulated strength of *multiple* affinities of individual noncovalent binding interactions) may dramatically improve targeting.

Numerous studies have also established additional correlations between particle size, complement activation, and phagocytic clearance [2]. For example, the extent of surface opsonization by C3b molecules and clearance kinetics by the mononuclear phagocyte system tends to increase with particle size when normalizing surface area. In accordance with the crystal structure of C3b, each surface-bound C3b molecule may occupy an area of $40\,nm^2$ on an NP surface [32]. With smaller particles, the bulk of activated C3 molecules will be released into the surrounding medium rather than deposited on the particle surface.

6.4 MACROPHAGE AVOIDANCE OF NANOPARTICLES

Surface strategies that generally suppress opsonization processes can limit particle recognition by macrophages. There are many examples from microbial systems as well as circulating cells such as erythrocytes that can be translated for design of "macrophage-resistant" particulate systems [5]. One approach is to minimize or eliminate complement activation (and hence complement fixation) [28,33]. Examples include surface modification or coating with naturally-occurring complement inhibitors [28,33]. Another strategy is to create a sufficient degree of steric barrier on the particle surface that can physically prevent particle interaction with macrophage receptors [5,34]. One approach is surface modification with methoxy poly(ethylene glycol), mPEG, and related macromolecules [1,2,5]. Macrophage-avoiding or stealth particles are typically below 150 nm in size, where the surface-projected PEG or related polymer chains provide stability to the particle suspension by repulsion through a steric mechanism of stabilization involving both enthalpic and entropic contributions [1,2,5]. Due to increased surface hydrophilicity and close association with water molecules, the steric barrier, and the structured water surrounding the barrier, may also suppress protein adsorption, but this does not necessarily prevent opsonization processes [34,35]. For instance, complement activation and fixation still proceeds with some surface-engineered particles where the extent of complement activation and fixation depends on surface density and conformation of the projected polymers [36,37]. The surface polymer conformational changes have further been shown to switch complement activation from one pathway to another [36,37]. The steric barrier on the NP surface, however, can interfere with the binding of C3b and/or iC3b to their corresponding macrophage receptors [34]. Stealth NPs have widely been used for passive targeting of selected pathological sites where anatomical openings exist (e.g., mostly sarcomas and to some extent certain carcinomas) [2,5].

Stealth particles may not necessarily avoid all macrophages. For example, splenic microcirculation (as in sinusoidal spleens) may direct certain stealth particles to the red-pulp macrophages as a result of efficient particle filtration at interendothelial cell slits in splenic venous sinuses [15]. Morphologically, these stealth particles are rigid nondeformable entities of 220−250 nm in diameter. Red-pulp macrophages in the vicinity of endothelial cell slits eventually take up filtered stealth NPs, but the mechanism of recognition remains unknown [38,39]. Newly-recruited macrophages. as well as activated macrophages. can also recognize some stealth particles independent of opsonization processes [5,35,40].

6.5 OTHER CHALLENGES

Complement activation and fixation remains a central point for efficient clearance and destruction of particulate invaders. However, inadvertent activation of the complement system may trigger consequential secondary responses with hemodynamic, respiratory, cutaneous, and subjective manifestations [41]. This is due to liberation of potent complement bioactive products (e.g., C3a, C5a, and C5b-9) with the ability to modulate the function of a variety of immune cells and vascular endothelial cells. For instance, excessive production of C5a may down-regulate immune responses in some leukocytes, while overactivating other cell types. Triggering of mast cells and basophils by anaphylatoxins may lead to secretion of a cocktail of vasoactive mediators (e.g., histamine, thromboxanes, leukotrienes) and induce anaphylaxis and other undesirable effects [41]. Finally, C5b-9 complexes may elicit nonlytic stimulatory responses from vascular endothelial cells and modulate endothelial regulation of hemostasis and inflammatory cell recruitment, whereas iC3b could induce up-regulation of certain adhesion molecules on neutrophils and endothelial cells.

The above-mentioned issues are of concern from a therapeutic angle because complement-related adverse reactions to various particulate carriers including stealth nanomedicines have been noted in the clinic [41,42].

REFERENCES

[1] Moghimi SM, Hunter AC, Murray JC. Nanomedicine: current progress and future prospects. FASEB J 2005;19:311–30.

[2] Moghimi SM, Hunter AC, Andresen TL. Factors controlling nanoparticle pharmacokinetics: an integrated approach and perspective. Ann Rev Pharmacol Toxicol 2012;52:481–503.

[3] Boraschi D, Costantino L, Italiani P. Interaction of nanoparticles with immunocompetent cells: nanosafety considerations. Nanomedicine (Lond) 2012;7:121–31.

[4] Dobrovolskaia MA, McNeil SE. Immunological properties of engineered nanomaterials. Nat Nanotechnol 2007;2:469–78.

[5] Moghimi SM, Hunter AC, Murray JC. Long-circulating and target-specific nanoparticles: theory to practice. Pharmacol Rev 2001;53:283–318.

[6] Moghimi SM, Parhamifar L, Ahmadvand D, Wibroe PP, Farhangrazi ZS, Hunter AC. Particulate systems for targeting of macrophages: basic and therapeutic concepts. J Innate Immun 2012;4:509–28.

[7] Torchilin VP. Recent advances with liposomes as pharmaceutical carriers. Nat Rev Drug Discov 2005;4:145–60.

[8] Pashine A, Vaiante NM, Ulmer JB. Targeting the innate immune responses with improved vaccine adjuvants. Nat Med 2005;11:S63–8.

[9] O'Hagan DT, Singh M, Ulmer JB. Microparticles for the delivery of DNA vaccines. Immunol Rev 2004;199:191–200.

[10] Moghimi SM. The innate immune responses, adjuvants and delivery systems. In: Jorgensen L, Nielsen HM, editors. Delivery technologies for biopharmaceuticals. Peptides, proteins, nucleic acids and vaccines. Chichester: Wiley; 2009. p. 113–27.

[11] Li H, Willingham SB, Ting JP, Re F. Cutting edge: inflammasome activation by alum and alum's adjuvant effects are mediated by NLRP3. J Immunol 2008;181:17–21.

[12] Taylor PP, Martinez-Pomares L, Stacey M, Lin H-H, Brown GD, Gordon S. Macrophage receptors and immune recognition. Annu Rev Immunol 2005;23:901–44.

[13] Sleyster EC, Knook DL. Relation between localization and function of rat liver Kupffer cells. Lab Invest 1982;47:484–90.

[14] Winkler G. Pulmonary intravascular macrophages in domestic animal species: a review of structural and functional properties. Am J Anat 1988;181:217–34.

[15] Moghimi SM. Mechanisms of splenic clearance of blood cells and particles: towards development of new splenotropic agents. Adv Drug Deliv Rev 1995;17:103–15.

[16] Moghimi SM. Exploiting bone marrow microvascular structure for drug delivery and future therapies. Adv Drug Deliv Rev 1995;17:61–73.

[17] Abu-Hijleh MF, Habbal OA, Moqattash ST. The role of the diaphragm in lymphatic absorption from the peritoneal cavity. J Anat 1995;186:453–67.

[18] Moghimi SM. Nanoparticle engineering for the lymphatic system and lymph node targeting. In: Broz P, editor. Polymer-based nanostructures. Medical applications. Cambridge: RSC Publishing; 2010. p. 81–97. RSC Nanoscience & Nanotechnology, No. 9

[19] Moghimi SM. Modulation of lymphatic distribution of subcutaneously injected poloxamer 407-coated nanospheres: the effect of the ethylene oxide chain configuration. FEBS Lett 2003;540:241–4.

[20] Moghimi SM. The effect of methoxy-PEG chain length and molecular architecture on lymph node targeting of immuno-PEG liposomes. Biomaterials 2007;27:136–44.

[21] Hunter AC, Elsom J, Wibroe PP, Moghimi SM. Polymeric particulate technologies for oral drug delivery and targeting: a pathophysiological perspective. Nanomedicine 2012;8(Suppl. 1):S5–20.

[22] Murray PJ, Wynn TA. Protective and pathogenic functions of macrophage subsets. Nat Rev Immunol 2011;11:723–37.

[23] Gordon S. Alternative activation of macrophages. Nat Rev Immunol 2003;3:23–35.

[24] Stoger JL, Goossens P, de Winther MPJ. Macrophage heterogeneity: relevance and functional implications in atherosclerosis. Curr Vasc Pharmacol 2010;8:233–48.

[25] Martinez FO, Gordon S, Locati M, Mantovani A. Transcriptional profiling of the human monocyte-macrophage differentiation and polarization: new molecules and patterns of gene expression. J Immunol 2006;177:7303–11.

[26] den Hann JMM, Kraal G. Innate immune functions of macrophage subpopulations in the spleen. J Innate Immun 2012;4:437–45.

[27] Tomita M, Yamamoto K, Kobashi H, Ohmoto M, Takao T. Immunohistochemical phenotyping of liver macrophages in normal and diseased human liver. Hepatology 1994;20:317–25.

[28] Moghimi SM, Andersen AJ, Ahmadvand D, Wibroe PP, Andresen TL, Hunter AC. Material properties in complement activation. Adv Drug Deliv Rev 2011;63:1000–7.

[29] Moghimi SM, Hunter AC. Recognition by macrophages and liver cells of opsonized phospholipid vesicles and phospholipid headgroups. Pharm Res 2001;18:1–18.

[30] Pedersen MB, Zhou X, Larsen EKU, Sørensen US, Kjems J, Nygaard JV, et al. Curvature of synthetic and natural surfaces is an important target feature in classical pathway complement activation. J Immunol 2010;184:1931–45.

[31] Barua S, Yoo J-W, Kolhar P, Wakankar A, Gokarn YT, Mitragotri S. Particle shape enhances specificity of antibody-displaying nanoparticles. Proc Natl Acad Sci USA 2013;110:3270–5.

[32] Janssen BJ, Christodoulidou A, McCarthy A, Lambris JD, Gros P. Structure of C3b reveals conformational changes that underlie complement activity. Nature 2006;444:213–6.

[33] Rodriguez PL, Harada T, Christian DA, Pantano DA, Tsai RK, Discher DE. Minimal "self" peptides that inhibit phagocytic clearance and enhanced delivery of nanoparticles. Science 2013;339:971–5.

[34] Moghimi SM, Hamad I, Andresen TL, Jørgensen K, Szebeni J. Methylation of the phosphate oxygen moiety of phospholipid-methoxy(polyethylene glycol) conjugate prevents PEGylated liposome-mediated complement activation and anaphylatoxin production. FASEB J 2006;20:2591–3.

[35] Moghimi SM, Szebeni J. Stealth liposomes and long circulating nanoparticles: critical issues in pharmacokinetics, opsonization and protein-binding properties. Prog Lipid Res 2003;42:463–78.

[36] Hamad I, Al-Hanbali O, Hunter AC, Rutt KJ, Andresen TL, Moghimi SM. Distinct polymer architecture mediates switching of complement activation pathways at the nanosphere-serum interface: implications for stealth nanoparticle engineering. ACS Nano 2010;4:6629–38.

[37] Andersen A, Robinson JT, Dai H, Andresen TL, Hunter AC, Moghimi SM. Single-walled carbon nanotube surface control of complement recognition and activation. ACS Nano 2013;7:1108–19.

[38] Moghimi SM, Porter CJH, Muir IS, Illum L, Davis SS. Non-phagocytic uptake of intravenously injected microspheres in rat spleen: influence of particle size and hydrophilic coating. Biochem Biophys Res Commun 1991;177:861–6.

[39] Moghimi SM, Hedeman IS, Muir IS, Illum L, Davis SS. An investigation of the filtration capacity and the fate of large filtered sterically-stabilized microspheres in rat spleen. Biochim Biophys Acta 1993;1157:233–40.

[40] Moghimi SM, Hedeman H, Christy NM, Illum L, Davis SS. Enhanced hepatic clearance of intravenously administered sterically stabilized microspheres in zymosan-stimulated rats. J Leukoc Biol 1993;54:513–7.

[41] Moghimi SM, Wibroe PP, Helvig SY, Farhangrazi ZS, Hunter AC. Genomic perspectives in inter-individual adverse responses following nanomedicine administration: the way forward. Adv Drug Deliv Rev 2012;64:1385–93.

[42] Moghimi SM, Farhangrazi ZS. Nanomedicine and complement paradigm. Nanomedicine 2013;9:458–60.

CHAPTER 7

The Invertebrate Immune System as a Model for Investigating the Environmental Impact of Nanoparticles

Laura Canesi[1] and Petra Procházková[2]

[1]DISTAV, Department of Earth, Environmental and Life Sciences, University of Genoa, Genoa, Italy
[2]Institute of Microbiology of the Academy of Sciences of the Czech Republic, Prague 4, Czech Republic

7.1 BRIEF OVERVIEW OF INVERTEBRATE IMMUNITY

Innate immunity is considered to be natural, nonspecific, nonanticipatory, and nonclonal, but germ line encoded; whereas adaptive immunity is indeed specific, anticipatory, clonal, and somatic [1,2] (Chapters 2 and 3). Invertebrates lack an adaptive immunity. However, over long periods of evolutionary time, millions of invertebrate species have developed many different defense strategies to successfully cope with invading bacterial, fungal, and viral pathogens, depending exclusively on innate immunity [1]. From the first Metchnikoff's observations of phagocytosis in different invertebrate and mammalian cells, suggesting an evolutionary mechanism devoted to protecting organisms from pathogen infections [2], a potent and complex innate immune system has been described in different invertebrate groups showing many commonalities to that of vertebrates [3,4].

Invertebrate systems rely on three basic mechanisms of immune defense: physicochemical barriers, cellular defenses, and humoral mechanisms (Figure 7.1), with cell and humoral responses acting in a coordinated way for efficient elimination of potential pathogens.

The common defense mechanisms used by most invertebrates are phagocytosis, production of reactive oxygen species (ROS) and nitrogen radicals, synthesis and secretion of antibacterial and antifungal proteins, cytokine-like proteins, hydrolytic enzymes, agglutination and nodule formation, encapsulation of foreign objects, activation of enzymatic cascades that regulate melanization and coagulation of hemolymph. These functions are generally carried out by free circulating

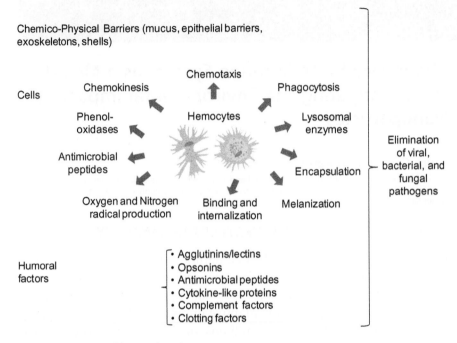

Figure 7.1 Components of the invertebrate immune system.

cells (hemocytes, coelomocytes) in the blood (hemolymph, coelomic cavity) (Figure 7.1). It should be noted, however, that in the nematode *Caenorhabditis elegans*, one of the invertebrate models most utilized for genetic and molecular studies on innate immunity, mobile immuno-cytes are not present, and intestinal epithelial cells are responsible for cell-mediated immune response [5].

Hyalinocytes, granulocytes, plasmatocytes, and coelomocytes are among the most common types of circulating cells identified in differ-ent invertebrate groups, with each species generally showing the pres-ence of different types of hemocytes (Table 7.1).

Distinct functions for each hemocyte type cannot be identified for all invertebrates, because a specific immune function (i.e., phagocyto-sis) performed by a morphological type of hemocyte in a particular species may be carried out by a different cellular type in another spe-cies. Despite the considerable efforts made for the characterization and classification of hemocytes, given the impressively wide diversity of their shapes and functions, the different methods and criteria used for their characterization, the lack of a defined hemopoietic organ in

Table 7.1 Examples of the Most Common Types of Invertebrate Immunocytes

Coelomocytes: heterogeneous morphology and functions, main immune cells in worms and echinoderms.

Granulocytes: include all hemocyte types filled with granules (basophilic, acidophilic) described in several invertebrates. Can perform different functions, from phagocytosis to encapsulation, in different species/taxa. Most similar to mammalian macrophages.

Hyalinocytes: agranular cells, molluscs (radical production) and crustaceans (clotting), phagocytosis.

Lamellocytes: large flat cells, encapsulation of large invading foreign material (insects).

Oenocytoids: main source of prophenoloxidases, enzymes required for melanization of invading organisms, as well as for wound repair (insects).

Plasmatocytes: small spherical hemocytes; phagocytosis, antimicrobial peptides, encapsulation (insects).

numerous organisms, and the inability to document cellular maturation, a comparison of these cells in different species, let alone in different taxa, is far from being established. However, regardless of this morphological and functional diversity, invertebrate immunocytes perform the same immune functions as vertebrate macrophages [6].

A wide range of molecules capable of recognizing pathogen-associated molecular patterns (PAMPs) common to many microorganisms, leading to activation of cell-mediated response, are present both on the hemocyte membrane and in hemolymph serum. Moreover, hemolymph serum contains a wide range of different secreted components that participate in agglutination, opsonization, degradation, encapsulation of microorganisms, as well as in clotting and wound healing [4,7].

The lack of acquired immunity and the capacity to form antibodies (specific response) does not mean lack of specificity: invertebrates have evolved genetic mechanisms capable of producing thousands of different proteins from a small number of genes; this diversity allows them to recognize and eliminate a wide range of different pathogens [8]. Among these, antimicrobial peptides (AMPs) are small cationic peptides with a remarkable structural diversity, engaged in the destruction of bacteria inside phagocytes, before being released into hemolymph to participate in systemic responses. AMPs appeared as one of the components of antimicrobial host defense throughout evolution [9].

Genetic and molecular studies carried out in model invertebrates (dipteran insect species and nematodes) lead to the identification of genes and proteins that play a key role in invertebrate immunity and greatly contributed to the knowledge of the molecular mechanisms of innate immunity in higher organisms. An example is the role discovered for the Toll pathway in the detection of microbial antigens and subsequent induction of innate immunity in Drosophila melanogaster [10,11] (Figure 7.2).

From the description of a number of conserved immune-related genes and related signaling pathways in D. melanogaster and C. elegans [12,13], research on immune diversity in different invertebrate species at the molecular level is becoming a central theme in the characterization of immune systems. Sequencing of genomes and transcriptomes of invertebrate species among cnidarians, worms, and echinoderms revealed an unexpected diversity of innate immune pathways. Several components which were thought to be restricted to the vertebrates were found to already occur in lower invertebrates and

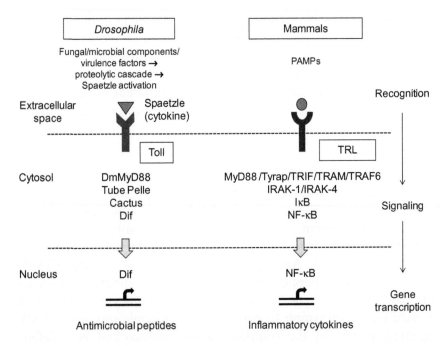

Figure 7.2 Simplified schematic representation of Toll/TLR pathways in Drosophila and mammals. Toll and TLRs activate an evolutionary conserved signaling pathway involving the Toll/interleukin-1R domain adapters DmMyD88 and MyD88, the kinases IRAK and Pelle, the inhibitors Cactus and IκB, and the Rel family transcription factors Dif and NF-κB. Mammalian TLRs are activated on direct binding of microbial molecular patterns, whereas Drosophila Toll is activated by the cytokine Spaetzle.

were lost or mutated beyond recognition during evolution in the classical invertebrate model organisms of insects and nematodes [14–16]. For example, genomes of *Drosophila* and *Caenorhabditis* lack components of the complement system, which previously led to the assumption that this pathway is restricted to the vertebrate system [15]. Other examples are amplification of the Toll receptor and the tumor necrosis factor (TNF) systems or the presence of components of the interferon regulatory factor family observed in lower invertebrates [16].

In general, analyses of newly available genome sequences, expressed sequence tag collections, and particular gene functions are providing a clearer picture and a more reliable estimate of the quality and amount of evolutionary changes occurring across the Metazoa [14–16]. Different species belonging to Anthozoa (corals) and Lophotrochozoa (annelids, molluscs) showed a significant better recovery of shared genes with humans (Deuterostomes) than with Ecdysozoa (nematodes, insects). These latter have high rates of molecular evolution and have suffered from major gene loss; this rapid genome change is likely to have occurred recently, and probably independently, in the fly and worm, associated with intense selection for small genome size, rapid developmental rates, and the highly specialized lifestyles [17].

With the progress of research on different invertebrate groups, an increasing number of genes, including antimicrobial peptides, components of the complement system, those involved in intracellular signal transduction of immune responses, extracellular C-type lectins, cytokine-like proteins, immunoglobulin domains, are being continuously discovered, revealing complex and sophisticated mechanisms of host defense [3,4]. These studies indicate that the most successful immune strategies have an early evolutionary origin and have probably been conserved over the billion years of separate evolution of invertebrates and vertebrates because of their high defensive value [18]. From studies on host defense systems at the genetic, molecular, and functional levels in invertebrates, we can learn about the fundamental conserved pathways, further expanding the general understanding of innate immunity [1,3,4].

The potential of invertebrate immunology does not rely only on conservation of the mechanisms of the immune response: other factors, such as environmental adaptation and life span of invertebrates, represent additional sources of information. Invertebrates represent about 95% of animal species, and are widespread in all types of environments, where they are subjected to a wide range of physical, chemical, and biological variables, including a complex microbiota that can represent an extensive attack of potential pathogens. As the immune system represents the physiological mechanism to ensure host survival in different habitats, invertebrate immunity provides an ideal model system for investigation of their response, and subsequent evolution of immune defenses, to cope with both natural and anthropogenic stressors in different environmental compartments [7,19]. The study of the immune response through traditional approaches, integrated with ecological, evolutionary, and population biology theories, led to the development of one of the most rapidly expanding fields of biology, "Ecological Immunology." Ecological immunology examines the impact of environmental stressors on the immune response, and in particular, how these stresses act to create and maintain the variation in the immune functions in the context of evolution and ecology [7,20].

It has been thought for a long time that the evolution of immune systems was needed to meet the requirements of an increasing life span, and that animals with only the innate immune system are simple and short lived. However, in comparison with classical invertebrate models for innate immunity (i.e., insects or worms), many invertebrate species (among them sea urchins, crustaceans, and molluscs) show a much longer long average life span (years). Others, like sponges and the freshwater polyp *Hydra*, are assumed to be nearly immortal [19]. Although studies directly linking immune responses and longevity are still scarce, recent investigations at the molecular level are providing indications about the complexity and diversification of the immune gene repertoire, which may contribute to the plasticity of immune responses in different long-lived invertebrates [3,21].

Overall, despite the common features in the mechanisms of innate immunity both at the functional and the molecular level, given the wide differences in invertebrate groups, their adaptation to different environments, and the enormous differences of life span, it is almost impossible to draw a general taxonomy of invertebrate immunity in an evolutionary context. However, the complexity of solutions displayed by different invertebrates to eliminate potential pathogens in the continuous arms race of host—microbe coevolution represents a wide and promising field for investigating different aspects of immune response.

The utilization of different invertebrate models offers significant advantages to the study of host—pathogen interactions, in particular the opportunity to study early infection processes, because not all interactions lead to disease. These interactions can also be investigated at different levels of organization: from the molecular approach, to *in vitro* and *in vivo* studies on circulating immunocytes, in many invertebrate species to the whole-organism level, in simpler, short lived, and thus genetically tractable model organisms (i.e., insects and nematodes). These approaches can be used in investigating responses to both natural pathogens for each species and to pathogens common to vertebrates and humans. This work appears to be promising in revealing common mechanisms of innate immunity, including the identification of universal defense genes and the pathways that control their expression in the response to infection.

7.2 INVERTEBRATE IMMUNITY AS A TARGET FOR ENVIRONMENTAL NANOPARTICLES

According to Baun et al. [22], invertebrate tests are well suited to generate reproducible and reliable nanotoxicity data to assess the environmental impact of manufactured nanomaterials or nanoparticles (NPs), due to the number and diversity of invertebrate species and their important role in different environments, as well as in the potential transfer of NPs through food chains. Apart from traditional ecotoxicity testing, it has been underlined how more specific assays, like immunotoxicity tests, may help understanding the major toxic mechanisms and modes of actions that could be relevant for different NP types in different organisms [23]. Conservation of the general mechanisms of innate immunity from invertebrates to mammals is a key feature that represents a useful basis for studying common biological responses to environmental contaminants, including NPs. However, given the heterogeneity of invertebrate immune systems, basic knowledge of the immune system of the model invertebrate used for testing the effects of environmental stressors, including NPs, is mandatory.

Research on the effects of NPs on the immune function in invertebrates is still in its infancy. Although immunotoxic effects of different types of NPs have been described in *Drosophila* [24], sea urchins [25], and polychaete worms [26,27], most available data so far are on bivalve molluscs and earthworms.

7.3 BIVALVE MOLLUSCS AS AN INVERTEBRATE MODEL FOR INVESTIGATING THE EFFECTS OF NANOPARTICLES ON INNATE IMMUNITY IN AQUATIC ENVIRONMENTS

7.3.1 Bivalve Immunity

Due to the continuous development and production of NPs, their uptake and effects in the aquatic biota represent a growing concern. Estuarine and coastal environments are expected to represent the ultimate sink for NPs, where their chemical behavior (aggregation/agglomeration) and consequent fate may be critical in determination of the biological impact [22]. Cell-mediated immunity and the phagocytic cells are being identified as the primary target of NPs in aquatic organisms [28].

Suspension-feeding invertebrates are particularly at risk of NP exposure, as they have extremely well developed systems for the uptake of nano- and microscale particles integral to key physiological functions such as intracellular digestion and cellular immunity [29]. Among these, bivalves (Mollusca, Lophotrochozoa) are a relevant ecological group, widespread in freshwater, estuarine, and marine environments, with many edible species, and widely utilized as sentinel organisms to evaluate the biological impact of different contaminants. Bivalve hemocytes are responsible for cell-mediated immunity through the combined action of the phagocytic process with humoral defense factors such as agglutinins (e.g., lectins), lysosomal enzymes (e.g., acid phosphatase, lysozyme), toxic oxygen intermediates, and various antimicrobial peptides [30]. Although bivalve hemocytes are extremely heterogeneous, in the marine mussel *Mytilus* spp. granular hemocytes represent the dominant cell type (Figure 7.3) and are considered mature cells being capable of phagocytosis, ROS and NO production, release of hydrolytic enzymes and antimicrobial peptides. Responses of mussel hemocytes to bacterial signals, cytokines, hormones, as well as to a variety of contaminants, have been largely characterized: in these cells, the immune function is modulated by conserved components of kinase-mediated cell signaling [31].

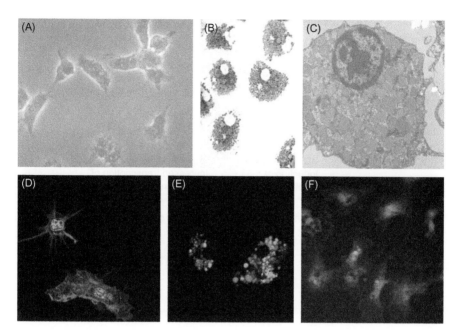

Figure 7.3 Representative images of Mytilus galloprovincialis *hemocytes. (A) Optical microscopy of unstained hemocytes and (B) Neutral-Red-stained lysosomes in granular hemocytes; (C) transmission electron microscopy of a mature granulocyte; (D, E) confocal fluorescence microscopy of hemocytes stained with (D) Alexa Fluor® 647 Phalloidin for actin (red) and Sybergreen for nuclei (green), (E) Lysotracker (green) for the lysosomal compartment. (For interpretation of the references to color in this figure legend, the reader is referred to the web version of this book.)* Kindly provided by C. Ciacci.

7.3.2 Effects of NPs in Bivalves

Increasing evidence supports the hypothesis that the immune function in bivalves represents a significant target for the effects of NPs (Figure 7.4). Although the first report of NP-induced immunomodulation *in vivo* was provided in the freshwater bivalve *Elliptio complanata* [32], the marine mussel *Mytilus* has been the species so far most utilized for studies on the effects and mechanisms of action of NPs on the immune function *in vitro* and *in vivo* (reviewed in Refs. [33–35]). *In vitro* studies showed that different NP types are rapidly taken up by *Mytilus galloprovincialis* hemocytes where they can affect a large number of functional parameters, from lysosomal function to phagocytic activity and oxyradical production, and also induce proapoptotic processes; the effects of NPs were mediated by stress-activated MAPK signaling, as in mammalian phagocytes (Figure 7.4) [33–35].

These studies, carried out in a range of concentrations (µg/ml) similar to those currently utilized for testing the responses to NPs in mammalian

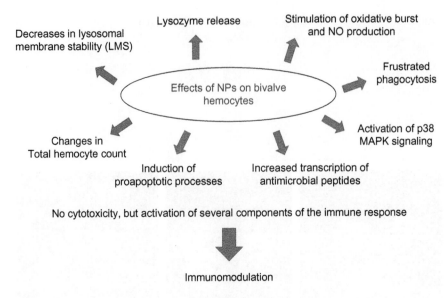

Figure 7.4 Summary of the in vitro *and* in vivo *effects of N Ps on bivalve hemocytes [33–35].*

cells, showed that the utilization of a battery of immunotoxicity tests in mussel hemocytes allows the rapid and sensitive evaluation of the *in vitro* effects of different types of NPs, from carbon-based NPs to *n*-metal oxides [34,35]. Another advantage of using bivalve hemocytes is that because bivalves have an open circulation, with blood often in direct contact with tissues, hemolymph can be drawn through simple, noninvasive methods (i.e., injection into the adductor muscle sinus). After sampling, animals can be reimmersed in water, where rapid recovery of hemolymph volume and circulating cells occurs. Overall, tests carried out in bivalve hemocytes proved a powerful tool for the rapid screening of the immunomodulatory effects of NPs, and they may represent robust alternative methods for testing chemicals within the REACH legislation (www.ec.europa.eu); moreover, their utilization may provide a basis for future experimental work for designing of environmentally safer nanomaterials. This approach has been recently applied in a pilot study for the screening of different NPs on the hemocytes of the oyster *Crassostrea gigas* [36]. The effects of *in vivo* exposure to different types of NPs have been investigated in different bivalve species, with effects mainly observed on lysosomal and oxidative stress parameters, and on apoptotic processes at the tissue level (mainly in gills and digestive gland), as well as on embryo development; distinct responses and tissue accumulation were detected depending on the NP type and on the concentration utilized [36].

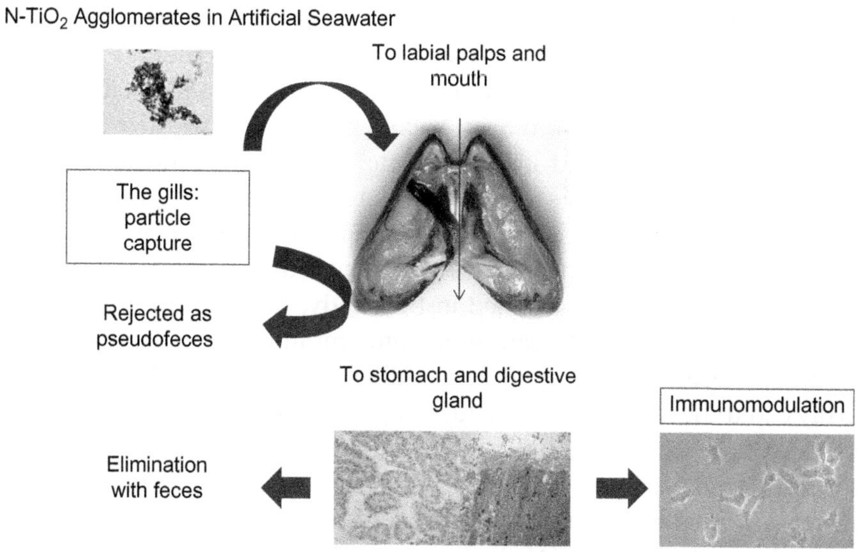

N-TiO$_2$ Agglomerates in Artificial Seawater

Figure 7.5 Possible pathways of in vivo *uptake of a model NP type (n-TiO$_2$) by* Mytilus *leading to immunomodulation. Particle agglomerates in seawater are taken up by the gills, entrapped in mucus, and rejected as pseudofeces or directed to labial palps and mouth. From labial palps, particles are directed toward the digestive system and to digestive cells in the hepatopancreas, where they can accumulate within the endolysosomal system or eliminated with feces. From the hepatopancreas, particles can pass into the circulatory system (hemolymph) to immune cells (hemocytes).*

In *Mytilus*, NPs showed immunomodulatory effects also *in vivo*. Exposure to different NPs [33,35], and in particular to *n*-TiO$_2$ utilized as a model NP [33,35], allowed formulating a hypothesis on the possible pathways leading to NP-induced immunomodulation (Figure 7.5).

Due to the physiological mechanisms involved in the feeding process, nano-TiO$_2$ agglomerates/aggregates formed in seawater are taken up by the gills and subsequently directed to the digestive gland, where intracellular uptake of nanosized materials induces lysosomal perturbations and changes in the expression of antioxidant genes and genes involved in the immune response (namely lysozyme and antimicrobial peptides) [33,35]. These results were obtained at NP concentrations much lower ($1-100$ μg/l) than those usually utilized in ecotoxicity tests on different aquatic organisms and closer to predicted environmental concentrations [22,23]. Nanosized particles can then be potentially translocated from the digestive system to the hemolymph, and to circulating hemocytes, where nano-TiO$_2$ induced changes in functional parameters, including lysosomal function, phagocytosis, ROS and NO (nitric oxide) production. Induction of preapoptotic processes was also observed at both the plasma membrane (annexin binding) and the mitochondrial level (changes in mitochondrial membrane potential and cardiolipin oxidation). Moreover, significant changes in the expression of antioxidant genes and immune-related genes, in particular antimicrobial peptides, were observed [33]. Interestingly, the effects of n-TiO$_2$ on expression of immune genes were opposite in the digestive gland (down-regulation) and hemocytes (up-regulation). Although a limited number of genes were examined in this study, these data represent the first evidence that NPs can modulate immune gene expression in bivalves. Recently, the rapidly expanding application of DNA microarrays and next-generation sequencing technologies offers new and broader research perspectives, from the whole transcriptome coverage to the *Mytilus* genome sequencing, leading to the identification of an increasing number of immune-related genes that could represent the target for different NPs [16,37,38]. Likely candidates are for example the members of the Toll receptor family recently identified in several bivalve species [16].

7.4 EARTHWORMS AS A MODEL FOR INVESTIGATING THE EFFECTS OF NANOPARTICLES ON INNATE IMMUNITY ON TERRESTRIAL INVERTEBRATES

7.4.1 Earthworm Immunity

Earthworms (Lumbricidae, Oligochaeta, Annelida) are mainly free-living terrestrial animals living in soil, leaf litter, under the stones, mainly in wetter, more heavily vegetated regions. As protostomian animals with a true coelom filled with coelomic fluid containing free coelomocytes, they have no lungs and breathe through the skin. For the gas exchange, it is necessary to keep the outermost layers moist by excretion of mucus onto the skin, which contains several antibacterial factors and thus represents the first protective barrier against invaders. Each segment of the cavity is interfaced with the outer environment by a dorsal pore enabling also the entering of the coelomic cavity by microorganisms. Therefore, the coelomic cavity is not aseptic and always contains bacteria, protozoa, and fungi from the outer environment. Earthworm skin with mucus is the first-line defense barrier against pathogens, but once they enter the coelom, they are exposed to cellular and humoral responses. The presence of phagocytes combined with humoral factors can easily prevent the coelomic bacteria from

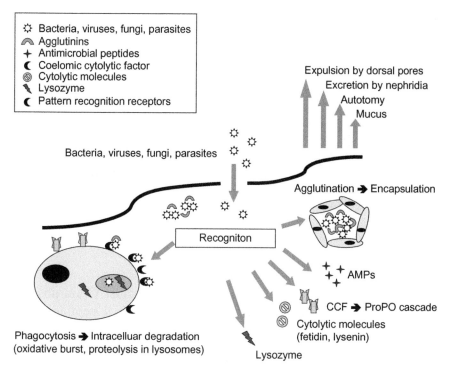

Figure 7.6 The general scheme of the innate defense of earthworms.

multiplying. Exhausted phagocytes can then be eliminated through dorsal pores. The attacking bacteria can be also excreted by nephridia, while large foreign bodies, agglutinated bacteria, or parasites can be eliminated by a process known as encapsulation (Figure 7.6) [39].

Earthworm coelomocytes are classified based on a differential stain-ing, ultrastructure, and granule composition (Figure 7.7) into two basic categories—amoebocytes (mainly immune function) and eleocytes (mainly nutritive function) [40]. The existence of self- and nonself-recognition in earthworms was proved already in the 1960s in trans-plantation experiments showing the response to the allografts as well as to xenografts [41], thus suggesting the occurrence of short-term and limited memory based only on cells (Figure 7.7) [42].

Among humoral defense mechanisms, one of many antimicrobial factors in earthworms is lysozyme that hydrolyze the 1,4-β-D-links between *N*-acetylmuramic acid and *N*-acetyl-D-glucosamine residues (GlcNAc) in the peptidoglycan of bacterial cell walls and thus

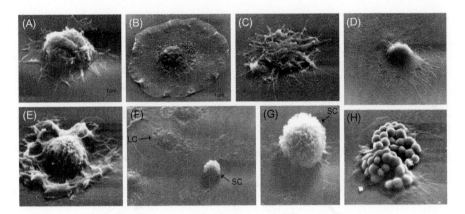

Figure 7.7 Immunocytes of earthworm Eisenia andrei *visualized by SEM. A−E—different types of adhered coelomocytes, F—free small coelomocyte (SC) and large coelomocyte (LC), G—small coelomocyte, H—coelomocyte-phagocyting glass beads.* Kindly provided by E. Kauschke.

efficiently contributes to the protection mainly against Gram-positive bacteria [43]. Only a limited number of antimicrobial peptides have been described in annelids; one of them, a proline-rich peptide named Lumbricin I, was isolated and characterized from *Lumbricus rubellus* [44]. The coelomic fluid of *Eisenia* earthworms exhibits numerous biological activities including bacteriostatic and bacteriolytic activities that are often connected with hemolytic activity. One group of characterized hemolytic and antimicrobial molecules is represented by fetidins [45] and lysenins [46], having antibacterial activity against both Gram-positive and Gram-negative bacteria. Moreover, these molecules are able to bind to sphingomyelin, a major lipid constituent of plasma membranes of most mammalian cells, where they polymerize and form channels through the lipid bilayer [47].

The recognition of microbial pathogens, as an essential element of the innate immune response, is mediated by pattern-recognition receptors (PRRs) recognizing molecular structures broadly shared by pathogens, known as PAMPs. The recognition of PAMPs by PRRs, like Toll-like receptors (TLRs), subsequently leads to the activation of signaling pathways resulting in the production of various inflammatory cytokines and antimicrobial peptides [48]. In annelids, TLRs were identified in the leeches *Helobdella robusta* and *Hirudo medicinalis*, and polychaete *Capitella capitata* [49,50].

Coelomic cytolytic factor (CCF) is a well-characterized 42-kDa lytic protein originally found in *Eisenia andrei*, acting in earthworm defense as a pattern-recognition molecule [51]. CCF is present on cells of the mesenchymal lining of the coelomic cavity as well as on free coelomocytes, and is also secreted into the coelomic fluid in a soluble form [52]. It shares functional analogies with the mammalian cytokine TNF based on similar saccharide-recognition specificity. CCF is formed by two spatially distinct lectin-like domains with the different binding specificities for PAMPs: one domain located in the central part of the molecule interacts with lipopolysaccharide (LPS) and β-1,3-glucans, and the second domain located in C-terminal part interacts with peptidoglycan constituents. Upon binding of PAMPs, CCF triggers the activation of the prophenoloxidase (proPO) cascade [53]. The proPO cascade is a sensitive and efficient defense system consisting of several proteins, such as zymogenic proteinases, proteinase inhibitors, proPO, PO, and PRRs with the final product melanin [54]. Melanin exhibits fungistatic, bacteriostatic, and antiviral properties and is involved also in wound healing and defense reaction. In earthworms, melanization reactions accompany the cellular defense reactions of the host, that is, encapsulation, resulting in the formation of so-called brown bodies.

7.4.2 Effects of NPs in Earthworms

Earthworms, constituting 60−80% of soil biomass, are widely used in standard toxicity tests for studies of soil pollution recommended by the International Organization for Economic Co-operation and Development and International Organization for Standardization. Earthworms appear to be suitable as biomonitoring organisms, particularly for their permanent direct contact with soil by both external and internal (intestinal lining) surfaces. Therefore, earthworms are effectively used in the research of nanomaterial interactions with living organisms and in assessing environmental nanosafety.

The widespread use of silver NPs leads to their release into the environment mainly through wastewater treatment plants as they enter the soil via biosolids or as the effluent from manufacturing processes. Hazards and risks of NPs exposure can be assessed at different endpoints. Profiles of proteins, metabolites, and gene expression represent rapid and sensitive responses of the organism to contaminant exposure. Endpoints at cellular level include induction of apoptosis, production of ROS, changes in mitochondrial membrane potential, reduction of ATP levels, production of cytokines, changes in phagocytic activity, and so on. Effects of NPs can be observed at the tissue level (histological changes), organism level (survival, growth, and reproduction), and population level (population growth rate and stage distribution).

In *Eisenia fetida, in vitro* exposure to Ag NPs induced accumulation of Ag NPs in coelomocytes, predominantly in a phagocytic population, with resultant oxidative stress and subsequent alteration of immune signaling [55]. Changes in the expression of nine stress response genes and in catalase activity [56], inhibition of glutathione reductase, acid phosphatase and Na^+, K^+-ATPase, were also described [57]. In contrast to a high accumulation of cobalt derived from Co NPs in the blood and the digestive tract, there were practically no Ag ions released and Ag NPs were excreted rapidly by earthworms essentially as intact particles [58].

In *Lumbricus terrestris, in vivo* exposure to nano-TiO_2 induced apoptotic processes. The highest apoptotic frequency was found in the cuticle, intestinal epithelium, and chloragogenous tissue, but no bioaccumulation of TiO_2 nanocomposites was observed, suggesting no permeation of these NPs into the coelom [59]. *In vitro* analysis in *E. fetida* showed that nano-TiO_2 was taken up by coelomocytes, and they could modify the molecular response of immune and detoxification system. Nano-TiO_2 caused an increase in fetidin and metallothionein (MT) messenger RNA (mRNA) expression, while the expression of CCF was decreased [60]. This study revealed that immune genes involved in defense mechanism appear to be very sensitive to nano-TiO_2 exposure. Furthermore, TiO_2 byproducts were shown to be bioaccumulated in earthworm tissue, to decrease phagocytosis, to increase expression of MT and superoxide dismutase mRNA, and to induce apoptosis [61]. NMR-based metabolomics as a more sensitive measure of *E. fetida* response to nano-TiO_2 in soil was used for detection of specific damage at the cellular or molecular level. This method revealed significant changes in metabolic profile consistent with oxidative stress as a proposed mechanism of toxicity [62]. Hu et al. showed that nano-TiO_2 as well as nano-ZnO could be accumulated in *E. fetida* and cause harmful effects such as oxidative stress, mitochondrial damage, biochemical and genotoxic responses, when its levels exceeded 1 g kg^{-1} in soil [63]. The dose of particles is one of the determining points for the reaction of immune system of the host. The toxicity of Cu NPs was tested mainly in enchytraeid *Enchytraeus albidus in vivo*, where induction of oxidative stress and differential gene expression were described. Moreover, microarray analysis revealed altered mRNA levels for specific genes mainly involved in metabolism, transcription, and translation or in the stress response, indicating oxidative stress conditions [64,65].

In vivo exposure of *L. rubellus* to fullerene NPs (C_{60}) in soil caused a reduction in growth and development [66]; sublethal concentrations of C_{60} also decreased gene expression of heat shock protein 70 and CCF. Moreover, earthworms exposed to C_{60} showed a damaged cuticle, with underlying pathologies of epidermis, muscles, and gut barrier [67]. This is in accordance with other findings, where coelomocytes exposed *in vitro* to C_{60} showed decreased gene expression of CCF, indicating immunosuppression [68]. On the other hand, in *E. fetida*, neither response of antioxidant enzyme expression or activity nor acute toxicity as a result of C_{60} occurrence in soil were detected [67,69].

Only a few papers exist about the toxicity of other types of NPs on earthworms. Different effects of nano-ZnO on *E. fetida*, including mortality, antioxidant enzyme activities, or accumulation of Zn in tissues, depending on the method of exposure, were described [70]. Nanosized zero-valent iron (nZVI) is used as a new remediation agent for contaminated soils, but it was shown that common field doses of nZVI have an acute adverse effect (reduced growth and reproduction, mortality), on both *E. fetida* and *L. rubellus* [71]. Also Au NPs were observed to cause untoward impact on *E. fetida* reproduction, and moreover, distribution of NPs in tissues of detritivores was demonstrated [72].

7.5 CONCLUSIONS

The increasing production and usage of nanosized products in various applications is followed by the necessity of assessing their safety for both humans and wildlife. Evaluating the interactions of NPs with the immune system is becoming an essential part of assessing nanosafety. The immune system is a dynamic network of cells, tissues, and organs that safeguard the body against attacks by invaders and protects against disease by identifying "self" and "nonself." NPs can be prepared to avoid immune system recognition, but when they are seen as foreign by the immune cells, it may result in a multilevel immune response. The interactions between NPs and the components of the immune system in wildlife are recently under intensive investigation. In this light, conservation of the main mechanisms of innate immunity from lower invertebrates to man may greatly help in understanding the possible interactions of NPs with the immune system. It has been shown in both aquatic and terrestrial models that various NPs can cause a broad scale of impacts, from slight changes of gene expression to the death of animals. The interactions of NPs with the immune system are influenced by many conditions, including the physicochemical characteristics of the particles (i.e., surface charge, NPs size, hydrophobicity, hydrophilicity, coatings) as well those of the receiving environment, routes of exposure in different cells and organisms. The utilization of invertebrate models also represents a promising field for designing environmentally, safer, "green" nanomaterials.

REFERENCES

[1] Kvell K, Cooper EL, Engelmann P, Bovari J, Nemeth P. Blurring borders: innate immunity with adaptive features. Clin Dev Immunol 2007;2007:83671.

[2] Cooper EL. Evolution of immune systems from self/not self to danger to artificial immune systems (AIS). Phys Life Rev 2010;7:55–78.

[3] Chang ZL. Recent development of the mononuclear phagocyte system: in memory of Metchnikoff and Ehrlich on the 100th anniversary of the 1908 Nobel Prize in Physiology or Medicine. Biol Cell 2009;101:709–21.

[4] Söderäll K. Invertebrate immunity. Advances in experimental medicine and biology. New York, NY: Landes Bioscience and Springer Science + Business Media, LCC; 2010. p. 314

[5] Marsh EK, May RC. *Caenorhabditis elegans*, a model organism for investigating immunity. Appl Environ Microbiol 2012;78:2075–81.

[6] Ottaviani E. Immunocyte: the invertebrate counterpart of the vertebrate counterpart of the vertebrate macrophage. Invertebr Surviv J 2011;8:1–4.

[7] Ellis P, Parry H, Spicer JI, Hutchinson TH, Pipe RK, Widdicombe S. Immunological function in marine invertebrates: responses to environmental perturbation. Fish Shellfish Immunol 2011;30:1209–22.

[8] Ghosh J, Lun CM, Majeske AJ, Sacchi S, Schrankel CS, Smith LC. Invertebrate immune diversity. Dev Comp Immunol 2011;35:959–74.

[9] Pasupuleti M, Schmidtchen A, Malmsten M. Antimicrobial peptides: key components of the innate immune system. Crit Rev Biotechnol 2012;32:143–71.

[10] Cooper EL, Kvell K, Engelmann P, Nemeth P. Still waiting for the toll? Immunol Lett 2006;104:18–28.

[11] Gilmore TD, Wolenski FS. NF-kappaB: where did it come from and why? Immunol Rev 2012;246:14−35.

[12] Hoffmann JA, Reichhart JM. *Drosophila* innate immunity: an evolutionary perspective. Nat Immunol 2002;3:121−6.

[13] Millet AC, Ewbank JJ. Immunity in *Caenorhabditis elegans*. Curr Opin Immunol 2004;16:4−9.

[14] Raible F, Arendt D. Metazoan evolution: some animals are more equal than others. Curr Biol 2004;14:R106−108.

[15] Kortschak RD, Samuel G, Saint R, Miller DJ. EST analysis of the cnidarian *Acropora millepora* reveals extensive gene loss and rapid sequence divergence in the model invertebrates. Curr Biol 2003;13:2190−5.

[16] Philipp EE, Kraemer L, Melzner F, Poustka AJ, Thieme S, Findeisen U, et al. Massively parallel RNA sequencing identifies a complex immune gene repertoire in the lophotrochozoan *Mytilus edulis*. PLoS One 2012;7:e33091.

[17] Perez DG, Fontanetti CS. Hemocitical responses to environmental stress in invertebrates: a review. Environ Monit Assess 2011;177:437−47.

[18] Boehm T. Evolution of vertebrate immunity. Curr Biol 2012;22:R722−732.

[19] Augustin R, Fraune S, Bosch TC. How *Hydra* senses and destroys microbes. Semin Immunol 2010;22:54−8.

[20] Rolff J, Siva-Jothy MT. Invertebrate ecological immunology. Science 2013;301:472−5.

[21] Rosenstiel P, Philipp EE, Schreiber S, Bosch TC. Evolution and function of innate immune receptors—insights from marine invertebrates. J Innate Immun 2009;1:291−300.

[22] Baun A, Hartmann NB, Grieger K, Kusk KO. Ecotoxicity of engineered nanoparticles to aquatic invertebrates: a brief review and recommendations for future toxicity testing. Ecotoxicology 2008;17:387−95.

[23] Crane M, Handy RD, Garrod J, Owen R. Ecotoxicity test methods and environmental hazard assessment for engineered nanoparticles. Ecotoxicology 2008;17:421−37.

[24] Galeone A, Vecchio G, Malvindi MA, Brunetti V, Cingolani R, Pompa PP. *In vivo* assessment of CdSe-ZnS quantum dots: coating dependent bioaccumulation and genotoxicity. Nanoscale 2012;4:6401−7.

[25] Falugi C, Aluigi MG, Chiantore MC, Privitera D, Ramoino P, Gatti MA, et al. Toxicity of metal oxide nanoparticles in immune cells of the sea urchin. Mar Environ Res 2012;76:114−21.

[26] Galloway T, Lewis C, Dolciotti I, Johnston BD, Moger J, Regoli F. Sublethal toxicity of nano-titanium dioxide and carbon nanotubes in a sediment dwelling marine polychaete. Environ Pollut 2010;158:1748−55.

[27] Cong Y, Banta GT, Selck H, Berhanu D, Valsami-Jones E, Forbes VE. Toxic effects and bioaccumulation of nano-, micron- and ionic-Ag in the polychaete, *Nereis diversicolor*. Aquat Toxicol 2011;105:403−11.

[28] Jovanovic B, Palic D. Immunotoxicology of non-functionalized engineered nanoparticles in aquatic organisms with special emphasis on fish-review of current knowledge, gap identification, and call for further research. Aquat Toxicol 2012;**118−119**:141−51.

[29] Moore MN. Do nanoparticles present ecotoxicological risks for the health of the aquatic environment? Environ Int 2006;32:967−76.

[30] Canesi L, Gallo G, Gavioli M, Pruzzo C. Bacteria-hemocyte interactions and phagocytosis in marine bivalves. Microsc Res Tech 2002;57:469−76.

[31] Canesi L, Betti M, Ciacci C, Lorusso LC, Pruzzo C, Gallo G. Cell signaling in the immune response of mussel hemocytes. Invertebr Surviv J 2006;3:40−9.

[32] Gagne F, Auclair J, Turcotte P, Fournier M, Gagnon C, Sauve S, et al. Ecotoxicity of CdTe quantum dots to freshwater mussels: impacts on immune system, oxidative stress and genotoxicity. Aquat Toxicol 2008;86:333−40.

[33] Barmo C, Ciacci C, Canonico B, Fabbri R, Cortese K, Balbi T, et al. *In vivo* effects of *n*-TiO$_2$ on digestive gland and immune function of the marine bivalve *Mytilus galloprovincialis*. Aquat Toxicol 2013;132-133:9−18.

[34] Ciacci C, Canonico B, Bilanicova D, Fabbri R, Cortese K, Gallo G, et al. Immunomodulation by different types of N-oxides in the hemocytes of the marine bivalve *Mytilus galloprovincialis*. PLoS One 2012;7:e36937.

[35] Canesi L, Ciacci C, Fabbri R, Marcomini A, Pojana G, Gallo G. Bivalve molluscs as a unique target group for nanoparticle toxicity. Mar Environ Res 2012;76:16−21.

[36] Abbott Chalew TE, Galloway JF, Graczyk TK. Pilot study on effects of nanoparticle exposure on *Crassostrea virginica* hemocyte phagocytosis. Mar Pollut Bull 2012;64:2251−3.

[37] Venier P, Varotto L, Rosani U, Millino C, Celegato B, Bernante F, et al. Insights into the innate immunity of the Mediterranean mussel *Mytilus galloprovincialis*. BMC Genomics 2011;12:69.

[38] Domeneghetti S, Manfrin C, Varotto L, Rosani U, Gerdo M, De Moro G, et al. How gene expression profiles disclose vital processes and immune responses in *Mytilus* spp. Invertebr Surviv J 2011;8:179−89.

[39] Ratcliffe NA, Rowley AF, Fitzgerald SW, Rhodes CP. Invertebrate immunity: basic concepts and recent advances. Internat Rev Cytol 1985;97:183−349.

[40] Sima P. Annelid coelomocytes and haemocytes: roles in cellular immune reactions. In: Vetvicka V, Sima P, Cooper EL, Bilej M, Roch P, editors. Immunology of annelids. Boca Raton, Ann Arbor, London, Tokyo: CRS Press; 1994. p. 11−165.

[41] Cooper EL, Roch P. Immunological profile of annelids: transplantation immunity. In: Vetvicka V, Sima P, Cooper EL, Bilej M, Roch P, editors. Immunology of annelids. Boca Raton, Ann Arbor, London, Tokyo: CRC Press; 1994. p. 201−43.

[42] Parry MJ. Survival of body wall autografts, allografts and xenografts in the earthworm *Eisenia foetida*. J Invert Pathol 1978;31:383−8.

[43] Joskova R, Silerova M, Prochazkova P, Bilej M. Identification and cloning of an invertebrate-type lysozyme from *Eisenia andrei*. Dev Comp Immunol 2009;33:932−8.

[44] Cho JH, Park CB, Yoon YG, Kim SC. Lumbricin I, a novel proline-rich antimicrobial peptide from the earthworm: purification, cDNA cloning and molecular characterization. Biochim Biophys Acta 1998;1408:67−76.

[45] Roch P, Valembois P, Davant N, Lassegues M. Protein analysis of earthworm coelomic fluid. II. Isolation and biochemical characterization of the *Eisenia foetida andrei* factor (EFAF). Comp Biochem Physiol 1981;69B:829−36.

[46] Sekizawa Y, Hagiwara K, Nakajima T, Kobayashi H. A novel protein, lysenin, that causes contraction of the isolated rat aorta: its purification from the coelomic fluid of the earthworm, *Eisenia foetida*. Biomed Res 1996;17:197−203.

[47] Shakor AB, Czurylo EA, Sobota A. Lysenin, a unique sphingomyelin-binding protein. FEBS Lett 2003;542:1−6.

[48] Janeway CA Jr., Medzhitov R. Innate immune recognition. Annu Rev Immunol 2002;20:197−216.

[49] Cuvillier-Hot V, Boidin-Wichlacz C, Slomianny C, Salzet M, Tasiemski A. Characterization and immune function of two intracellular sensors, HmTLR1 and HmNLR, in the injured CNS of an invertebrate. Dev Comp Immunol 2011;35:214–26.

[50] Davidson CR, Best NM, Francis JW, Cooper EL, Wood TC. Toll-like receptor genes (TLRs) from *Capitella capitata* and *Helobdella robusta* (*Annelida*). Dev Comp Immunol 2008;32:608–12.

[51] Bilej M, Brys L, Beschin A, Lucas R, Vercauteren E, Hanusova R, et al. Identification of a cytolytic protein in the coelomic fluid of *Eisenia foetida* earthworms. Immunol Lett 1995;45:123–8.

[52] Bilej M, Rossmann P, Sinkora M, Hanusova R, Beschin A, Raes G, et al. Cellular expression of the cytolytic factor in earthworms *Eisenia foetida*. Immunol Lett 1998;60:23–9.

[53] Bilej M, De Baetselier P, Van Dijck E, Stijlemans B, Colige A, Beschin A. Distinct carbohydrate recognition domains of an invertebrate defense molecule recognize Gram-negative and Gram-positive bacteria. J Biol Chem 2001;276:45840–7.

[54] Söderhäll K, Cerenius L, Johansson MW. The prophenoloxidase activating system and its role in invertebrate defence. Ann N Y Acad Sci 1994;712:155–61.

[55] Hayashi Y, Engelmann P, Foldbjerg R, Szabo M, Somogyi I, Pollak E, et al. Earthworms and humans *in vitro*: characterizing evolutionarily conserved stress and immune responses to silver nanoparticles. Environ Sci Technol 2012;46:4166–73.

[56] Tsyusko OV, Hardas SS, Shoults-Wilson WA, Starnes CP, Joice G, Butterfield DA, et al. Short-term molecular-level effects of silver nanoparticle exposure on the earthworm, *Eisenia fetida*. Environ Pollut 2012;171:249–55.

[57] Hu C, Li M, Wang W, Cui Y, Chen J, Yang L. Ecotoxicity of silver nanoparticles on earthworm *Eisenia fetida*: responses of the antioxidant system, acid phosphatase and ATPase. Toxicol Environ Chem 2012;94:732–41.

[58] Coutris C, Hertel-Aas T, Lapied E, Joner EJ, Oughton DH. Bioavailability of cobalt and silver nanoparticles to the earthworm *Eisenia fetida*. Nanotoxicology 2012;6:186–95.

[59] Lapied E, Nahmani JY, Moudilou E, Chaurand P, Labille J, Rose J, et al. Ecotoxicological effects of an aged TiO$_2$ nanocomposite measured as apoptosis in the anecic earthworm *Lumbricus terrestris* after exposure through water, food and soil. Environ Int 2011;37:1105–10.

[60] Bigorgne E, Foucaud L, Caillet C, Giambérin L, Nahmani J, Thomas F, et al. Cellular and molecular responses of *E. fetida* coelomocytes exposed to TiO$_2$ nanoparticles. Nanopart Res 2012;14:959.

[61] Bigorgne E, Foucaud L, Lapied E, Labille J, Botta C, Sirguey C, et al. Ecotoxicological assessment of TiO$_2$ byproducts on the earthworm *Eisenia fetida*. Environ Pollut 2011;159:2698–705.

[62] Whitfield Aslund ML, McShane H, Simpson MJ, Simpson AJ, Whalen JK, Hendershot WH, et al. Earthworm sublethal responses to titanium dioxide nanomaterial in soil detected by (1)H NMR metabolomics. Environ Sci Technol 2012;46:1111–8.

[63] Hu CW, Li M, Cui YB, Li SS, Chen J, Yang LY. Toxicological effects of TiO$_2$ and ZnO nanoparticles in soil on earthworm *Eisenia fetida*. Soil Biol Biochem 2010;42:586–91.

[64] Gomes SI, Novais SC, Gravato C, Guilhermino L, Scott-Fordsmand JJ, Soares AM, et al. Effect of Cu-nanoparticles versus one Cu-salt: analysis of stress biomarkers response in *Enchytraeus albidus* (*Oligochaeta*). Nanotoxicology 2012;6:134–43.

[65] Gomes SI, Novais SC, Scott-Fordsmand JJ, De Coen W, Soares AM, Amorim MJ. Effect of Cu-nanoparticles versus Cu-salt in *Enchytraeus albidus* (*Oligochaeta*): differential gene expression through microarray analysis. Comp Biochem Physiol C Toxicol Pharmacol 2012;155:219−27.

[66] van der Ploeg MJ, Baveco JM, van der Hout A, Bakker R, Rietjens IM, van den Brink NW. Effects of C60 nanoparticle exposure on earthworms (*Lumbricus rubellus*) and implications for population dynamics. Environ Pollut 2011;159:198−203.

[67] van der Ploeg MJ, Handy RD, Heckmann LH, van der Hout A, van den Brink NW. C(60) exposure induced tissue damage and gene expression alterations in the earthworm *Lumbricus rubellus*. Nanotoxicology 2013;7:432−40.

[68] van der Ploeg MJ, van den Berg JH, Bhattacharjee S, de Haan LH, Ershov DS, Fokkink RG, et al. *In vitro* nanoparticle toxicity to rat alveolar cells and coelomocytes from the earthworm *Lumbricus rubellus*. Nanotoxicology 2012;: doi: 10.3109/17435390.2012.744857

[69] Li D, Alvarez PJ. Avoidance, weight loss, and cocoon production assessment for *Eisenia fetida* exposed to C(6)(0) in soil. Environ Toxicol Chem 2011;30:2542−5.

[70] Li LZ, Zhou DM, Peijnenburg WJ, van Gestel CA, Jin SY, Wang YJ, et al. Toxicity of zinc oxide nanoparticles in the earthworm, *Eisenia fetida* and subcellular fractionation of Zn. Environ Int 2011;37:1098−104.

[71] El-Temsah YS, Joner EJ. Ecotoxicological effects on earthworms of fresh and aged nano-sized zero-valent iron (nZVI) in soil. Chemosphere 2012;89:76−82.

[72] Unrine JM, Hunyadi SE, Tsyusko OV, Rao W, Shoults-Wilson WA, Bertsch PM. Evidence for bioavailability of Au nanoparticles from soil and biodistribution within earthworms (*Eisenia fetida*). Environ Sci Technol 2010;44:8308−13.

CHAPTER 8

Summary and Outlook

Albert Duschl

Department of Molecular Biology, University of Salzburg, Salzburg, Austria

8.1 THE ROLE OF IMMUNITY IN NANOSAFETY

The previous chapters have elaborated the special role of immunology in nanosafety assessment: due to its ability to sense nonself and to respond to danger signals with vigorous defense mechanisms, the immune system is ideal for monitoring of potential early reactions toward nanomaterials. Innate immunity has evolved to respond very quickly to threats, as microbial pathogens can multiply exponentially once they have colonized the body. A very fast defense is therefore of utmost importance for survival, because slower reactions may be overwhelmed by the sheer number of microorganisms, and the body may already be too much weakened to survive the infection. The evolutionary advantage of fast immune responses is clear, and indeed the first components of innate immunity are already found in single-cell eukaryotes like amoeba [1] and, in more developed forms, key components of innate immunity are present in all multicellular organisms (Chapter 7) [2].

These characteristics imply that in particular the innate immunity can provide early readouts. Changes in protein expression, for example, secretion of cytokines and chemokines, are easily detected. The earliest secreted proteins are detectable within $1-2$ h by standard technologies like ELISA. Some effects on signaling pathways and gene expression are detectable within minutes after stimulation. Importantly, reactions of innate immunity usually occur much earlier and at much lower stimulus concentrations than cell death, an event that is assayed by a variety of tests that measure either viable cells or dead cells. Thinking about the safety profile of a novel material, we would like to know at what point detrimental changes occur, which may be much earlier than the lethal dose for cells or organisms. Some aspects cannot be properly addressed by immunological endpoints, for instance genotoxicity, so additional methods are always required. However, we know that immune responses provide early warning signs, including cell stress that is induced along with the start of innate reactions. In any case, it is important to distinguish between a simple reaction, which is a sign of recognition of nonself and therefore a normal "physiological" defense activity, and a prepathological detrimental response, such as a response that does not resolve with time or is too intense or persists too long. If detrimental responses are detected only at concentrations that are much higher than any reasonable scenario for human exposure would suggest, then the material should be considered as safe according to the best available knowledge.

Immunity has evolved mechanisms for recognizing very specifically nonself-entities associated with danger, along with the ability to maintain an "immunological memory" throughout life. These mechanisms, which are collectively called adaptive immunity, are found in vertebrates, down to the level of teleost (bony) fish [3]. These adaptive mechanisms respond slower and take several days to develop. First signals may by readable after 1−2 days. Even if those readouts—secreted and membrane-bound proteins, along with changes in transcriptome, metabolome, and specific signaling pathways—are slower than innate reactions, they contain valuable additional information. The immune system can respond in different ways, and at the interface between innate and adaptive immunity we find the answers to a crucial issue: some hallmarks of inflammation and cell stress are induced under conditions that fall well within the range of a normal environment. We will then observe fluctuations that are part of the body's main function, which is to maintain homeostasis. If we observe massive release of pro-inflammatory cytokines initiated by innate immune mechanisms, we are looking at a full defensive response that indicates imminent danger. In contrast, very low levels of mediators may be considered to be insignificant, reflecting a minor response to a harmless stimulus. Where is the border between these two situations? That is hard to define for readouts of the innate immune system, but it can often be clearly stated for adaptive immunity.

One of the functions of adaptive immunity is to ensure tolerance against stimuli that have been assessed and were classified as harmless. Finding anergic T cells, or, more easily, regulatory T cells (Tregs) induced by a particular nanomaterial indicates an active effort not to react to a harmless substance. Regulatory T cells can be characterized by markers like the transcription factor FoxP3 and—technically simpler—by secretion of the immunosuppressive cytokines, IL-10 and

TGF-β, which are detectable for example by ELISA. The establishment of tolerance implied by the differentiation of Tregs would be considered the best available proof the immune system considers a specific type of nanoparticle (NP) as being not dangerous.

On the other hand, if a dangerous entity should be present, the innate immune mechanisms create a milieu that favors the development of type-1 immune responses, associated with specific T cell subsets (T_H1, T_H17, T_H22). Allergic reactions, using type-2 immune responses, are characterized by T_H2 and probably T_H9 cells. All these cell types can be identified and their development gives us specific information about the ongoing response. In cases of an active immune response, examining adaptive reactions thus provides insights into the defensive mechanisms that are invoked, which may in turn help to identify the features of the nanomaterial that led to immunotoxicity.

8.2 CHALLENGES FOR THE FURTHER DEVELOPMENT OF THE FIELD

If you ask immunologists about the most irritating problems in their practical work with nanomaterials, the contamination of samples will probably be close to the top of the list [4,5]. Immune cells are exquisitely sensitive to bacterial compounds, and it is very difficult to reliably exclude those ubiquitous materials. Testing for lipopolysaccharide (LPS) is only part of the answer because many other bacterial compounds are also powerful stimuli for immune cells, but in contrast to LPS there is usually no commercial assay available to test for them. LPS can be destroyed by heating to 250°C, but many materials will not stand that kind of treatment. Even if a batch of NPs has been rendered totally free of bacterial products, it may be a problem to keep them out during transport, storage, and handling. It is an acute problem to distinguish true NP effects from those of bystander substances.

The contamination issue leads to the development of refined protocols that imply the use of rigorously purified NPs. This is a valuable approach for work toward understanding the mechanisms of interaction between NPs and biological entities, but as methods get more and more refined, they get less and less able to work with real-life particles that are not ultraclean. More elaborate methods are also less likely to be suitable for testing large numbers of samples. The latter would be important to deal for example with batch-to-batch variability of NPs, which can be quite substantial. One would sometimes want to test every batch of NPs at least with some quick tests and, considering the large number of samples that it may be desirable to test, such tests should also be robust and affordable. Reporter genes induced by promoters activated in cell stress and early immune reactions are an example of suitable models for medium-to-high throughput formats and still give information on relevant endpoints for the assessment of nanosafety [6–8]. The technical development of the field is thus moving in two different directions: more elaborate techniques are designed to understand the *bona fide* interactions between NPs and cells at a mechanistic level, and more robust assays are developed to deal with large numbers of samples that are not clean and contain a mixture of NPs and other types of materials. For materials collected on-site, it is likely that engineered NPs will constitute only a fraction of the total material, so it is a challenge to develop protocols that allow, under such conditions, assessing NP effects specifically.

Considering on-site situations, for example, in the workplace, chronic and repeated exposure have to be taken into account. It is essentially impossible to assess this properly with cell culture methods. Even well-maintained cultures of primary cells deteriorate after a few weeks, while with continuous cell lines the risk of accidental contamination is high due to the frequent manipulation of the cultures that is necessary to keep the cells alive. In case of a contamination with bacteria or yeasts or mycoplasmas, the culture has to be discarded. Even if no such accidents occur, a few weeks of tests are not accurately reflecting the situation of workplace exposure that may go on for years.

Exposure of laboratory animals would be theoretically an alternative, but the large number of mice or rats needed as sentinels is raising ethical issues. A specific ethical problem is that for on-site exposure it would not be clear which endpoints are relevant. Indeed, because for many endpoints mouse inflammatory responses may significantly differ from those in humans, knowing the endpoints is mandatory for establishing the relevance of the animal models [20]. Thus, planning animal experiments without a real hypothesis is a clear violation of the 3R principle, besides risking to be useless or, even worse, misleading. In addition, maintaining for example a rodent colony over years is expensive, and we cannot expect that many people in the workforce would be cheerful about mice or rats kept next to them, even if it is done for monitoring their own workplace safety.

The evolutionary ancient roots of the immune system allow another perspective. Many responses are evolutionarily conserved, so it may be possible to use invertebrates for monitoring purposes [1,3]. Environmental science has developed many models that allow following the development of small invertebrates over many generations. It would be interesting to compare conserved immune parameters in such invertebrates. These models are cheap and do not raise ethical problems, and in addition there are suitable organisms both for terrestrial and aquatic exposure, as elaborated in Chapter 7. For assessing chronic and repeated exposure, using invertebrates is an interesting perspective.

8.3 UNDERSTANDING MOLECULAR MECHANISMS

The most desired situation is to avoid altogether producing nanomaterials that may cause problems through the implementation of "safety-by-design" procedures. In order to do this, it is important not only to correctly identify the existence of a problem but also to understand the molecular mechanisms that are responsible for the problem observed, eventually correlating them with the NP features [9]. Ideally, it may then be possible to re-engineer the materials in such a way that their desired features are maintained while the problematic aspects are lost.

Understanding the molecular mechanisms underlying the observed toxicity of some nanomaterials will be crucial to further progress of the field. NPs may be carriers of other substances (like LPS or chemicals carried over from synthesis), they may dissolve in the body into potentially dangerous compounds like metal ions and, in case of long and stiff fibers, fiber toxicity related to frustrated phagocytosis, oxidative stress, and apoptosis may be induced [10,11]. Rather specific for some NPs is their ability to induce production of reactive oxygen species (ROS) at their surface [12–14]. Immune mechanisms play a role in several recognized pathways (cell stress induced by toxic compounds, frustrated phagocytosis, ROS production, etc.), but often it is not understood why the immune system responds to some types of NPs. This uncertainty is reflected in conflicting literature reports, of which many examples have been quoted in the previous chapters. In these cases, it is usually not clear why different results are obtained even with allegedly identical nanomaterials. Many different explanations may be suggested, including slight but crucial differences in nanomaterials used, contamination with various agents, aging processes, different cell lines and biological materials, time points of measurement, etc. The high variability of NPs encounters high variability of the biological test systems. For example, even if the same stable cell line was used it cannot be taken for granted that the cells will react the same way in different laboratories. Culture conditions and media may vary, cell lines are often mislabeled [15] and, even if they are correctly identified, cells of the same cell line propagated in different laboratories may have individual properties due to genetic drift.

How to get out of that quagmire? While rigorous controls at every step help to reduce problems, the only real solution is an improved understanding of the molecular mechanisms that mediate interactions between NPs and the immune systems. If it is known that a specific receptor gets activated and that such activation is related to health problems, it is possible to test directly for the activation of that receptor and ignore much of the other events. The situation is similar to the case of carcinogens, where a clear understanding is gained only when the mechanism of action is understood. The same applies to immune reactions.

We know a lot about the molecular mechanisms that lead to breach of tolerance against pathogens and parasites. Sensing of bacterial or viral compounds via pattern-recognition receptors is well understood, and the recognition of endogenous danger signals released, for example, by necrotic cells is also an established paradigm. We know that specific peptides and antigen structures are recognized by T cells and by B cells, respectively, resulting in powerful adaptive immune reactions. For some particles, activation of inflammasomes has been shown, and it is recognized that this depends, for example, in the case of carbon nanotubes, on their functionalization [16]. Studies of this type have the potential to link very specific features of nanomaterials with equally specific features of immune components. An increased understanding of the molecular mechanisms involved in these interactions will allow developing quick tests for evaluating the most crucial endpoints, to implement safety-by-design strategies, and to suggest new paradigms for the medical application of nanomaterials for suppressing, activating, or modifying immunity.

8.4 APPLYING NANOTECHNOLOGY IN IMMUNOLOGY

An immediate benefit of nanotechnology is that it enables immunologists to learn more about the immune system. Nanosized particles have been around since the beginning of life, and distinguishing harmless dust from dangerous viral particles of the same size has been a perpetual task of the immune system. In particular, we can expect to learn more about the mechanisms for establishing tolerance, as this will usually be the best response when abiotic nanosized particles are encountered.

A recent cover of *Nature Reviews Immunology* (August 2013) featured the topic "Immunological applications of nanotechnology" [17], so the immunological community is fully aware of the exciting new possibilities deriving from these new materials. The greatest interest is created not by questions of nanosafety—so far a more niche type of topic—but by the desire to develop new tools for preventive and therapeutic applications. Immunomodulatory effects of NPs can result in immune activation (mostly in the form of inflammation) but they can also lead to immunosuppression. Both pathways are eagerly followed up.

Immune activation by abiotic materials is a key feature of adjuvants, and using NPs in adjuvant formulations for improved efficacy is a major area of research right now. The adjuvant effect is clearly desired for vaccination, but it can also be exploited when NPs are used as drug carriers. For example, stimulating certain types of inflammatory processes helps to destroy cancers [18]. A nanodrug that carries a cytostatic agent could as well provide immunoactivating signals at the same time: two very different antitumor effects from the same drug, which may be synergistic for therapy.

Immune suppression is a major issue in autoimmunity, allergy, and in transplant patients. Existing immunosuppressive treatments are successful but not satisfactory, because they generally suppress immunity rather broadly, with the collateral effect of putting patients at risk of

Table 8.1 NPs and the Immune System

- NPs mostly fail to trigger an immune response (lack of recognition, active immunological tolerance)
- NPs may induce an inflammatory immune response (both innate and adaptive) against themselves and against adsorbed proteins (foreign molecules, modified self-proteins) in some circumstances
- Immune responses triggered by NPs do not result always in pathology (resolution of the response is the normal outcome)
- NPs may contribute to persistent inflammation and tissue destruction, with pathological consequences, in some circumstances
- Assessing NP interaction with the immune system can provide sensitive and relevant endpoints for detecting early reaction
- Exploiting NPs for modulating immune responses is the most promising avenue of nanomedicine:
  - inducing localized inflammatory reaction to amplify immunogenicity of vaccines (adjuvant effect)
  - inducing high-dose tolerance to autoimmunity-associated peptides
  - selectively suppressing or enhancing phagocyte effector functions (e.g., in inflammatory diseases vs. tumors)

infections. In addition, when the doses used are/become insufficiently effective, this results in loss of tolerance and organ rejection. More powerful or more specific immunosuppressants are among the drugs under development in nanomedicine. For instance, induction of tolerance against autoimmunity-causing self-peptides by delivering high doses of them with NPs is among the goals of achieving specific immunosuppression of the autoimmune reaction without having the side effects of general immunosuppression [19].

We can expect in the future that nanotechnological developments will contribute to the progress of immunological research and to its application for preventing and curing disease (Table 8.1). It is to be hoped that immunology can also aid the progress of nanotechnology, by providing suitable methods for identifying hazardous compounds early on in product development, and by helping to monitor NP effects to ensure safety of workers, consumers, and the environment.

REFERENCES

[1] Escoll P, Rolando M, Gomez-Valero L, Buchrieser C. From amoeba to macrophages: exploring the molecular mechanisms of *Legionella pneumophila* infection in both hosts. Curr Top Microbiol Immunol 2013. Available from: http://dx.doi:10.1007/82_2013_351.

[2] Paul WE. Fundamental immunology. Philadelphia, PA: Wolters Kluwer/Lippincott Williams & Wilkins; 2008.

[3] Boehm T. Design principles of adaptive immune systems. Nat Rev Immunol 2011;11:307–17.

[4] Oostingh GJ, Casals E, Italiani P, Colognato R, Stritzinger R, Ponti J, et al. Problems and challenges in the development and validation of human cell-based assays to determine nanoparticle-induced immunomodulatory effects. Part Fibre Toxicol 2011;8:8.

[5] Pfaller T, Colognato R, Nelissen I, Favilli F, Casals E, Ooms D, et al. The suitability of different cellular *in vitro* immunotoxicity and genotoxicity methods for the analysis of nanoparticle-induced events. Nanotoxicology 2010;4:52−72.

[6] Oostingh GJ, Schmittner M, Ehart AK, Tischler U, Duschl A. A high-throughput screening method based on stably transformed human cells was used to determine the immunotoxic effects of fluoranthene and other PAHs. Toxicol In Vitro 2008;22:1301−10.

[7] Herzog E, Byrne HJ, Davoren M, Casey A, Duschl A, Oostingh GJ. Dispersion medium modulates oxidative stress response of human lung epithelial cells upon exposure to carbon nanomaterial samples. Toxicol Appl Pharmacol 2009;236:276−81.

[8] Kohl Y, Oostingh GJ, Sossalla A, Duschl A, von Briesen H, Thielecke H. Biocompatible micro-sized cell culture chamber for the detection of nanoparticle-induced IL8 promoter activity on a small cell population. Nanoscale Res Lett 2011;6:505.

[9] Donaldson K, Murphy F, Schinwald A, Duffin R, Poland CA. Identifying the pulmonary hazard of high aspect ratio nanoparticles to enable their safety-by-design. Nanomedicine (Lond) 2011;6:143−56.

[10] Schinwald A, Donaldson K. Use of back-scatter electron signals to visualise cell/nanowires interactions *in vitro* and *in vivo*; frustrated phagocytosis of long fibres in macrophages and compartmentalisation in mesothelial cells *in vivo*. Part Fibre Toxicol 2012;9:34.

[11] Murphy FA, Schinwald A, Poland CA, Donaldson K. The mechanism of pleural inflammation by long carbon nanotubes: interaction of long fibres with macrophages stimulates them to amplify pro-inflammatory responses in mesothelial cells. Part Fibre Toxicol 2012;9:8.

[12] Kovacic P, Somanathan R. Nanoparticles: toxicity, radicals, electron transfer, and antioxidants. Methods Mol Biol 2013;1028:15−35.

[13] Syed S, Zubair A, Frieri M. Immune response to nanomaterials: implications for medicine and literature review. Curr Allergy Asthma Rep 2013;13:50−7.

[14] Fubini B, Ghiazza M, Fenoglio I. Physico-chemical features of engineered nanoparticles relevant to their toxicity. Nanotoxicology 2010;4:347−63.

[15] Capes-Davis A, Theodosopoulos G, Atkin I, Drexler HG, Kohara A, MacLeod RA, et al. Check your cultures! A list of cross-contaminated or misidentified cell lines. Int J Cancer 2010;127:1−8.

[16] Yang M, Flavin K, Kopf I, Radics G, Hearnden CH, McManus GJ, et al. Functionalization of carbon nanoparticles modulates inflammatory cell recruitment and NLRP3 inflammasome activation. Small 2013. Available from: http://dx.doi:10.1002/smll.201300481.

[17] Smith DM, Simon JK, Baker Jr. JR. Applications of nanotechnology for immunology. Nat Rev Immunol 2013;13:592−605.

[18] Coussens LM, Zitvogel L, Palucka AK. Neutralizing tumor-promoting chronic inflammation: a magic bullet?. Science 2013;339:286−91.

[19] Getts DR, Martin AJ, McCarthy DP, Terry RL, Hunter ZN, Yap WT, et al. Microparticles bearing encephalitogenic peptides induce T cell tolerance and ameliorate experimental autoimmune encephalomyelitis. Nat Biotechnol 2012;30:1217−24.

[20] Seok J, Warren HS, Cuenca AG, Mindrinos MN, Baker HV, et al. The Inflammation and Host Response to Injury, Large Scale Collaborative Research Program. Genomic responses in mouse models poorly mimic human inflammatory diseases. Proc Natl Acad Sci USA 2013;110:3507−12.

GLOSSARY

Adaptive immunity   the complex of defensive immune activities that are antigen-specific. Adaptive immunity develops slower than innate immunity, but achieves much higher selectivity and forms an immunological memory. Upon re-infection, an antigen can be cleared faster.

Alarmin   a danger signal for the immune system resulting from the own body, often a DAMP.

Anergy   a state in which a T cell becomes permanently inactivated, induced by an episode of insufficient stimulation.

Antibody   soluble or membrane-bound proteins that can bind two identical antigens. They are produced by B cells and are the mainstay of many processes in adaptive immunity. Numerous antibodies are used as medical drugs, due to the high specificity which they achieve.

Antigen   every entity that can be specifically recognized by antibodies or antigen receptors.

APC   antigen-presenting cells (APCs) are dendritic cells, macrophages, and B cells. They express MHC-II and can activate adaptive immunity.

Apoptosis   programmed cell death, a normal and frequent event in the body. No danger signals are released, in contrast to necrosis.

B cell/B lymphocyte   cell of the adaptive immune system that upon antigen triggering and specific T-cell help becomes a plasma cell that is producing antigen-specific antibodies.

Cell stress   a fixed set of cellular responses that are induced by any perceived disturbance (physical, chemical, and biological) via a wide variety of sensors. Cell stress reactions aim at re-establishing cellular homeostasis.

Complement   a set of blood proteins that can induce inflammation and kills targets by forming holes in bacterial membranes. Antibody-coated bacteria are particularly attacked by complement. The process does not require immune cells but is mediated entirely by blood proteins.

Cytokine   the cytokines are soluble proteins that are used for communication of immune cells with each other and with tissue cells. Examples include various interleukins, interferons, and growth factors.

DAMP   danger-associated molecular patterns (DAMPs) are signals produced by the body that indicate acute damage. Many DAMPs are released by cells dying during necrosis.

Dendritic cell (DC)   leukocyte population specialized in antigen presentation. DC can be a differentiation stage of monocytes and are often the first cells to recognize nonself, which results in activation of adaptive immune responses.

Immunogen   every entity that is able to raise a specific immune response. An immunogen is also an antigen, whereas the reverse is not true.

Immunoglobulin   synonym for antibody.

Inflammasome   a protein complex of somewhat variable composition that is formed in immune cells upon sensing of serious alarm signals. Inflammasome formation leads to the production of active pro-inflammatory and fever-inducing cytokines.

Inflammation   classically defined by reddening, swelling, pain, increased temperature, and reduced function. These symptoms are mediated by innate immunity. The swelling, for example, is due to immune cells that migrate to a site of infection.

Innate immunity   the complex of nonspecific rapid defensive immune reactions relying on pathogen recognition by a fixed set of receptors that are active from birth. It is often used as synonym for inflammation. However, some adaptive immune mechanisms can also contribute to inflammation as well.

Leukocyte   white cell of the blood. Leukocytes include mononuclear and polymorphonuclear phagocytes, lymphocytes, dendritic cells, and NK cells.

Lymphocyte   a class of mononuclear immune cells belonging to the adaptive immune system. Lymphocytes include T (thymus-derived) and B (bursa-derived) cells that upon antigen activation differentiate into a variety of specific effector cells.

Macrophage   highly phagocytic cells in tissues with many functions, including elimination of pathogens, antigen presentation, and removal of debris. Several subsets can be distinguished, which are adapted to functions in specific tissues.

MHC   a membrane protein complex that occurs in two versions: MHC-I is produced on all nucleated body cells. It contains peptides derived from the proteins that are produced by the cell. Appearance of unusual peptides indicates deviation, for example, virus infection or tumor formation. Such cells are destroyed by cytotoxic T cells. MHC-II is produced only by antigen-presenting cells. Here the peptide contained in the MHC complex is derived from entities taken up by the presenting cell. Nonself-peptides can stimulate adaptive immunity by activating T-Helper cells.

Monocyte   an immune cell in the blood that can efficiently take up invaders, like bacteria, but, in contrast to the neutrophil, is long lived. Ingested microorganisms get digested.

Necrosis   violent and unplanned death of a cell, usually resulting in the release of DAMPs, which lead to activation of innate immunity.

Neutrophil   an important effector cell in innate immunity that is especially suited to take up and kill bacteria. Pus is mostly neutrophils that have eaten themselves to death with bacteria.

NK   natural killer. NK cells are innate effector cells that can recognize anomalous cells (e.g., tumor cells) and kill them.

PAMP   pathogen-associated molecular patterns (PAMPs) are structures shared by many bacteria or viruses. They are recognized by specific receptors that trigger inflammation.

Pentraxins   serum proteins with various functions. In immunity they recognize PAMPs and activate inflammation processes.

Phagocyte   specialized innate immune cell able to ingest and degrade foreign material; phagocytes in humans include mononuclear phagocytes (monocytes and macrophages) and polymorphonuclear leukocytes (neutrophils or PMN).

PMN   an abbreviation that stands for polymorphonuclear leukocyte or neutrophil.

Polymorphonuclear cell   or polymorphonuclear leukocyte, one of the two types of phagocytic leukocytes in the blood, which extravasates and enters the affected tissue in situations of damage or infection.

ROS   an abbreviation that stands for reactive oxygen species, produced by activated phagocytes, have potent microbiocidal and membrane-damaging capacity.

T cell/T lymphocyte   a lymphocyte derived from thymus, which upon activation can functionally differentiate into antigen-specific T-helper, T-cytotoxic, and T-memory cells.

TLR   Toll-like receptor, a class of innate receptors structurally related to the *Drosophila* Toll molecule. In man, there are 10 TLRs that recognize different ranges of molecular patterns.

Printed and bound by CPI Group (UK) Ltd, Croydon, CR0 4YY

03/10/2024

01040426-0014